AF212737

Contemporary Challenges in Postnatal Care

Edited by Tanya Connell

Published in London, United Kingdom

Contemporary Challenges in Postnatal Care
http://dx.doi.org/10.5772/intechopen.104333
Edited by Tanya Connell

Contributors
Tripti Sinha, Ejura Ochala, Amen A. Bawazir, Juliana Yartey Enos, Samuel Kweku Enos, Edem Magdalena Tette, Richard Dickson Amoako, Beatrice Offeibea Hayford, Nur Intan Kusuma, Siti Khuzaiyah, Rini Kristiyanti, Lia Dwi Prafitri, Suparni Suparni, Nur Chabibah, Tanya Connell

© The Editor(s) and the Author(s) 2024

The rights of the editor(s) and the author(s) have been asserted in accordance with the Copyright, Designs and Patents Act 1988. All rights to the book as a whole are reserved by INTECHOPEN LIMITED. The book as a whole (compilation) cannot be reproduced, distributed or used for commercial or non-commercial purposes without INTECHOPEN LIMITED's written permission. Enquiries concerning the use of the book should be directed to INTECHOPEN LIMITED rights and permissions department (permissions@intechopen.com).

Violations are liable to prosecution under the governing Copyright Law.

Individual chapters of this publication are distributed under the terms of the Creative Commons Attribution 3.0 Unported License which permits commercial use, distribution and reproduction of the individual chapters, provided the original author(s) and source publication are appropriately acknowledged. If so indicated, certain images may not be included under the Creative Commons license. In such cases users will need to obtain permission from the license holder to reproduce the material. More details and guidelines concerning content reuse and adaptation can be found at http://www.intechopen.com/copyright-policy.html.

Notice

Statements and opinions expressed in the chapters are these of the individual contributors and not necessarily those of the editors or publisher. No responsibility is accepted for the accuracy of information contained in the published chapters. The publisher assumes no responsibility for any damage or injury to persons or property arising out of the use of any materials, instructions, methods or ideas contained in the book.

First published in London, United Kingdom, 2024 by IntechOpen
IntechOpen is the global imprint of INTECHOPEN LIMITED, registered in England and Wales, registration number: 11086078, 5 Princes Gate Court, London, SW7 2QJ, United Kingdom

British Library Cataloguing-in-Publication Data
A catalogue record for this book is available from the British Library

Additional hard and PDF copies can be obtained from orders@intechopen.com

Contemporary Challenges in Postnatal Care
Edited by Tanya Connell
p. cm.
Print ISBN 978-1-83768-224-9
Online ISBN 978-1-83768-225-6
eBook (PDF) ISBN 978-1-83768-775-6

We are IntechOpen, the world's leading publisher of Open Access books

Built by scientists, for scientists

6,800+
Open access books available

183,000+
International authors and editors

195M+
Downloads

156
Countries delivered to

Our authors are among the
Top 1%
most cited scientists

12.2%
Contributors from top 500 universities

WEB OF SCIENCE™

Selection of our books indexed in the Book Citation Index in Web of Science™ Core Collection (BKCI)

Interested in publishing with us?
Contact book.department@intechopen.com

Numbers displayed above are based on latest data collected.
For more information visit www.intechopen.com

For EU product safety concerns:
IN TECH d.o.o., Prolaz Marije Krucifikse Kozulić 3, 51000 Rijeka, Croatia,
info@intechopen.com or visit our website at intechopen.com.

Meet the editor

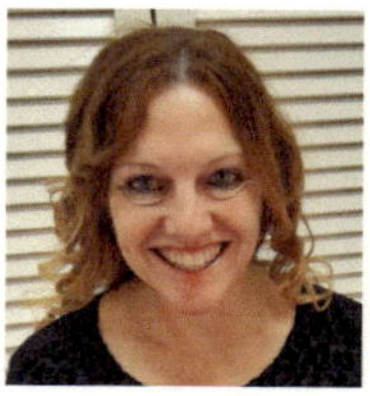

Dr. Tanya Connell studied nursing at the University of Technology Sydney, Australia, and midwifery at Western University, Sydney, Australia. She worked as a private maternity nurse/nanny/singer in England and Germany for 2 years. She worked as a midwife at various hospitals while studying to be a child and family health nurse, childbirth educator, and lactation consultant. Dr. Connell obtained a master's degree in Adult Education in 2004. She also has an MSc and Ph.D. She was recently a Senior Lecturer in Nursing at Auckland University of Technology, New Zealand, before moving back to Australia. Dr. Connell's passion is ensuring that all women have perinatal mental health assessment, screening, and services.

Contents

Preface

This book presents a global perspective on contemporary challenges in postnatal care.

Chapter 1, "Perspective Chapter: Psychosocial Screening and Assessment in the Private Sector in Australia during the Postnatal Period", is a perspective chapter discussing psychosocial screening and assessment in the postnatal period in the private sector in Australia. Postnatal mental health issues have long-term effects on families. Rates of maternal death by suicide are highest in the first year after giving birth. Thus, it is essential to screen and assess women for mental health issues. Women with mental health issues need to be identified early and referred to services to enhance their chance of an optimal outcome for their family. A sustainable model is essential to ensure that an appropriate healthcare professional identifies risks/concerns and engages with women who decline assistance. Timely postnatal psychosocial screening and assessment for private sector women is crucial, but barriers exist. This chapter discusses possible solutions to these challenges.

Chapter 2, "Barriers and Challenges in the Acceptance and Continuation of Postpartum Intrauterine Contraceptive Device", focuses on barriers and challenges in the acceptance of intrauterine contraceptive devices (IUCDs). These devices range from temporary birth-spacing methods to permanent birth-limiting methods. Despite the advantages of these devices, the acceptance and long-term uptake of IUCDs are lacking, and thus, have little impact on fertility rates in countries that would benefit from such. This is due to provider and logistical barriers in addition to family views. Although the uptake of IUCDs is insufficient for lowering total fertility rates, it is a relevant option for women. However, information, education, and communication (IEC) strategies, counseling, insertion training, and addressing prejudices about devices are needed.

Chapter 3, "Perspective Chapter: Contemporary Challenges in Postnatal Care in Low- and Middle-Income Countries", discusses neonatal and maternal burdens in low- and middle-income countries. There is a need to enhance maternal well-being and support newborn care, as maternal and neonatal mortality remains high. This objective aligns with the World Health Organization's Sustainable Development Goals, which are hoped to be achieved by the end of 2030. The chapter discusses strategies to reach a positive postnatal outcome, barriers to achieving this outcome, and unmet needs for family planning related to poor postpartum education. Strengthening health systems is essential to improve optimal care for families. These include infrastructure, equipment, water, sanitation, energy, and staff. Postnatal care affects the facility, household, and community levels.

Chapter 4, "Breastfeeding by Mothers with Cesarean Section Delivery", discusses Cesarean section deliveries and their association with lower breastfeeding rates. This is partly due to the separation of mother and baby, delay in early initiation of breast-feeding, and lack of milk supply. Therefore, a Cesarean delivery is an obstacle to early breastfeeding initiation. Healthcare providers must provide education to mothers to encourage them to breastfeed or to have a normal delivery to enhance their chances of breastfeeding.

Chapter 5, "Addressing Postnatal Challenges: Effective Strategies for Postnatal Care", highlights how mothers undergo numerous physical, economic, psychological, and sociological changes after giving birth. Challenges of motherhood include the decision to breastfeed, perinatal medical conditions and complications, and more. This chapter presents strategies for addressing postnatal challenges as well as strategies to improve patient information management, organizational standards, and protocols and policies. The chapter also examines the role of the midwife in postpartum care. Health organizations and regulatory bodies need to provide leadership to achieve a safe healthcare system and ensure an adequate work environment to provide competent quality care that promotes maternal well-being.

Chapter 6, "Perspective Chapter: Challenges to Postnatal Care in Sub-Saharan Africa – A Review", examines the postnatal period and the associated risk of neonatal and maternal mortality. Essential care for the family is needed to improve family mortality and morbidity. However, access to essential perinatal care is challenging, especially in resource-limited settings. This chapter highlights challenges to postnatal care in sub-Saharan Africa, where uptake of postnatal care is lacking, resulting in high postnatal neonatal and maternal morbidity mortality rates. Challenges include limited healthcare infrastructure, poor access to basic health services, poverty, cultural practices, illiteracy, marginalization of women, and political issues. Innovative approaches are needed to increase postnatal care provision to improve access and usage of postnatal care in the area, improve maternal and child health outcomes, and ultimately achieve the Sustainable Development Goals by 2023. Women in sub-Sahara Africa must be empowered economically and socially and provided with education, improved healthcare infrastructure, trained healthcare professionals, and high-quality postnatal care.

I would like to thank the authors for their contributions.

Dr. Tanya Connell
The University of Sydney,
Sydney, Australia

Section 1

Barriers

Chapter 1

Perspective Chapter: Psychosocial Screening and Assessment in the Private Sector in Australia during the Postnatal Period

Tanya Connell

Abstract

This chapter is a perspective literature review of published policy and literature regarding psychosocial screening and assessment in the postnatal period. The postnatal period is considered from birth until 6 weeks postpartum. This chapter focuses on the postnatal period, although some resources discussed are for women perinatally. Psychosocial assessment allows the identification of circumstances that affect a woman's mental health. Postnatal mental health is a contemporary challenge as its risks have long-term effects on the mother, infant and their family. The first year postpartum has the highest rate of maternal death by suicide, especially between nine and 12 months postpartum. Postnatally, the peak rate of hospitalisation for mental illness is within the first 3 months postpartum. The greatest risk for incident hospital admission specifically for primiparous women is 10–19 days postpartum. Psychosocial screening and assessment in the postnatal period are recommended internationally. However, in the private sector in Australia this is at the discretion of the private healthcare providers (postnatal midwife, child and family health nurse, obstetrician, paediatrician). Considering the potentially high morbidity related to postnatal mood disorders, it is crucial that women, either at risk or symptomatic of maternal depression and anxiety, be identified as early as possible in the postnatal period and be subsequently referred for appropriate local management.

Keywords: mothers, neonatal, care, obstetric, postnatal

1. Introduction

1.1 Postnatal mental health

Postnatal mental ill-health refers to any mental health condition affecting the mood, behaviour, well-being and/or daily function of a new parent. Perinatal mental health affects around 100,000 families across Australia every year. Postnatal mental health disorders are increasingly prevalent; however, some mothers do manage, with varying degrees of support. Phua et al. [1] results showed that positive antenatal mental health

IntechOpen

was uniquely associated with the children's cognitive, language and parentally rated competences, indicating that the effects of positive maternal mental health are likely to be distinct from only the absence of symptoms of depression or anxiety.

Internationally, postpartum depression is prevalent in 17% of the world's maternal population in 80 countries (see **Table 1**) [2]. In high-income countries (HICs), the prevalence of postnatal depression is reported to be 1:10 women. In low-middle-income countries, these prevalence rates are higher (19% during the postnatal period). The higher prevalence rates of maternal depression are often related to

Subgroup	Studies	Prevalence		PPD	Participants	*P* value	I^2
Country						<0.01	
South Africa	6	38.79	(25.71–53.72)	1076	3144		98.00%
Malawi	3	13.57	(8.94–20.07)	116	830		77.50%
Zambia	1	9.71	(6.74–13.79)	27	278		
Ghana	4	8.00	(1.90–28.13)	606	4294		99.30%
Cote d'Ivoire	1	14.13	(10.90–18.11)	51	361		
Egypt	6	22.99	(12.99–37.38)	472	2218		97.50%
Sudan	2	7.56	(5.47–10.34)	35	467		0.00%
Zimbabwe	2	27.22	(16.52–41.41)	281	1137		94.80%
Ethiopia	13	22.79	(18.07–28.33)	2666	11,534		97.50%
Tanzania	3	12.30	(11.22–13.49)	407	3310		98.00%
Nigeria	7	17.93	(10.19–29.59)	1008	10,659		0.00%
Israel	12	12.90	(9.38–17.50)	1188	9158		96.60%
Japan	27	13.30	(12.25–14.41)	25,035	199,089		96.20%
India	14	18.81	(13.59–25.44)	1817	10,554		97.60%
Turkey	26	21.87	(18.12–26.15)	3038	12,370		96.30%
Malaysia	6	12.64	(6.97–21.86)	1021	10,402		98.80%
China	42	17.98	(15.32–20.99)	5946	31,517		97.10%
Taiwan	17	21.65	(17.56–26.38)	661	3141		88.00%
Vietnam	8	13.77	(8.54–21.47)	1009	7314		98.20%
Pakistan	3	35.45	(18.47–57.10)	440	1326		97.60%
United Arab Emirates	1	18.31	(10.94–29.03)	13	71		—
Nepal	11	16.41	(12.07–21.91)	538	2443		92.80%
Thailand	8	12.52	(8.02–19.01)	514	4547		96.10%
Singapore	6	14.24	(10.10–19.71)	402	2602		98.40%
Bangladesh	10	26.65	(20.00–34.56)	1329	4423		98.80%
Qatar	3	18.00	(16.90–19.16)	795	4417		91.70%
USA	66	18.56	(16.91–20.34)	34,380	242,105		96.70%
Canada	25	13.89	(11.43–16.79)	13,421	118,968		98.60%
Australia	23	11.22	(9.23–13.56)	6928	82,680		0.00%

Subgroup	Studies	Prevalence		PPD	Participants	*P* value	I2
Argentina	2	29.88	(19.30–43.14)	165	625		83.00%
France	8	14.63	(10.01–20.89)	493	3203		93.80%
Oman	2	16.38	(9.15–27.58)	160	874		90.60%
Brazil	31	20.51	(18.53–22.65)	19,960	88,955		98.00%
Poland	5	17.91	(9.19–31.97)	365	2013		97.60%
Spain	5	9.09	(6.97–11.78)	360	3704		84.10%
UK	13	21.50	(17.63–25.94)	25,786	219,769		98.40%
Sweden	14	12.18	(9.41–15.63)	2057	18,189		97.20%
Kuwait	1	11.72	(10.11–13.55)	158	1348		—
Norway	12	11.24	(8.31–15.03)	1711	12,557		97.00%
Iran	18	24.41	(17.18–33.43)	5834	15,753		99.20%
Kenya	3	25.20	(11.50–46.63)	70	391		90.50%
Jordan	4	39.78	(21.43–61.54)	539	1333		98.20%
Uganda	1	32.67	(27.60–38.18)	98	300		—
Indonesia	2	11.76	(3.73–31.43)	51	440		93.90%
Eswatini	1	47.37	(38.39–56.52)	54	114		—
Syria	1	28.24	(25.66–30.96)	312	1105		—
Saudi Arabia	7	20.08	(14.17–27.65)	457	2305		93.40%
New Zealand	5	10.58	(5.62–19.01)	681	8057		98.30%
Multi	3	20.21	(10.16–36.19)	233	1474		96.60%
Morocco	1	27.00	(19.22–36.51)	27	100		—
Subgroup	Studies	Prevalence		PPD	Participants	*P* value	I2
Portugal	4	18.28	(12.57–25.81)	115	663		77.90%
Italy	14	16.79	(11.63–23.64)	1283	10,800		97.70%
Netherlands	7	10.69	(5.76–18.98)	1222	13,069		99.10%
Ireland	3	11.14	(10.13–12.25)	1275	11,694		19.10%
Iraq	1	28.40	(25.69–31.28)	284	1000		—
Greece	4	12.26	(8.02–18.30)	155	1259		83.40%
Hungary	1	16.54	(12.54–21.50)	44	266		—
Lebanon	1	12.75	(8.28–19.13)	19	149		—
Korea	4	22.50	(12.01–38.17)	246	1263		96.10%
Finland	3	14.62	(9.83–21.20)	320	2513		92.20%
Denmark	2	6.48	(5.70–7.36)	219	3381		0.00%
Czech Republic	2	15.82	(7.08–31.66)	59	408		90.30%
Belgium	1	23.94	(15.44–35.19)	17	71		—
Philippines	1	16.36	(11.47–22.81)	27	165		—
Mexico	1	20.00	(15.13–25.96)	42	210		—
Hong Kong	4	16.96	(13.77–20.70)	321	1860		71.90%
Greenland	1	8.62	(5.26–13.81)	15	174		—

Subgroup	Studies	Prevalence		PPD	Participants	*P* value	I^2
Germany	3	9.76	(5.26–17.40)	161	1760		92.90%
Bahrain	1	37.13	(31.21–43.46)	88	237		—
Serbia	3	23.66	(10.41–45.27)	134	573		95.60%
Peru	1	29.97	(28.00–32.02)	597	1992		—
Armenia	2	14.08	(11.48–17.14)	82	583		0.00%
Mongolia	1	9.10	(7.50–11.00)	95	1044		—
Russia	2	13.54	(1.71–58.45)	205	820		97.80%
Switzerland	1	21.93	(17.39–27.27)	59	269		—
Croatia	1	45.03	(37.74–52.54)	77	171		—
Slovenia	1	31.82	(19.84–46.81)	14	44		—
Afghanistan	1	60.93	(54.25–67.22)	131	215		—
Chile	3	28.27	(14.87–47.08)	177	629		95.10%
Timor-Leste	1	25.29	(19.33–32.36)	43	170		—
Jamaica	1	34.25	(24.31–45.79)	25	73		—
Continent						<0.01	
Southern Africa	7	39.96	(27.81–53.48)	1130	3258		97.70%
Eastern Africa	26	20.21	(16.86–24.04)	3665	17,780		97.00%
Western Africa	12	13.62	(8.27–21.62)	1665	25,314		99.00%
Northern Africa	9	18.75	(11.40–29.26)	534	2785		96.90%
Western Asia	62	19.83	(17.33–22.58)	7133	34,950		97.20%
Eastern Asia	96	17.39	(16.09–18.77)	32,429	238,273		97.70%
Southern Asia	56	22.32	(18.48–26.70)	9964	35,227		98.80%
Southeastern Asia	33	13.53	(11.00–16.52)	3208	26,677		97.30%
Northern America	92	17.01	(15.68–18.44)	47,816	361,247		98.70%
Oceania	28	11.11	(9.27–13.25)	7609	90,737		98.30%
South America	37	21.71	(19.78–23.76)	20,899	92,201		97.80%
Western Europe	20	12.91	(9.44–17.40)	1952	18,372		97.90%
Eastern Europe	10	16.62	(10.95–24.43)	673	3507		96.50%
Northern Europe	47	13.78	(12.47–15.21)	31,368	268,103		97.20%
Southern Europe	31	16.34	(12.90–20.48)	1997	16,177		96.60%
Central America	1	20.00	(15.13–25.96)	42	210		96.70%
Caribbean	1	34.25	(24.31–45.79)	25	73		—
Multiple	3	20.21	(10.16–36.19)	233	1474		—
Development						<0.01	
Developing	295	19.99	(18.76–21.27)	54,145	266,334		98.30%
Developed	276	14.85	(14.22–15.51)	118,197	970,031		98.20%
Country or regional income						<0.01	
High	314	15.54	(14.90–16.20)	121,333	985,634		98.20%
Upper-middle	178	19.68	(18.26–21.19)	41,217	186,768		98.40%

Subgroup	Studies	Prevalence		PPD	Participants	P value	I2
Lower-middle	56	20.14	(16.39–24.50)	5769	39,108		98.50%
Low	23	20.02	(15.32–25.73)	4023	24,855		98.70%
Publication date						0.58	
Before 2010	145	17.94	(15.79–20.30)	19,417	120,264		98.80%
After 2010	426	17.28	(16.54–18.05)	152,925	1,116,101		98.80%
Study size						≤0.01	
<1000	421	19.44	(18.40–20.51)	27,433	137,934		95.70%
>1000	150	12.97	(12.03–13.96)	144,909	1,098,431		99.50%
Diagnostic technique						<0.01	
DSM-IV	7	12.94	(9.14–18.00)	378	3086		91.50%
SRQ	12	25.90	(21.16–31.27)	3681	12,948		97.70%
PHQ-9	19	18.59	(12.21–27.44)	2475	23,846		99.10%
EPDS	464	16.86	(16.04–17.72)	110,611	775,287		98.70%
CES-D	13	25.06	(19.55–31.50)	2763	19,702		97.80%
BDI	10	29.70	(23.07–37.31)	553	1767		89.30%
DASS	4	18.47	(16.43–20.70)	1234	6863		72.40%
SCID	5	10.11	(3.75–24.48)	1712	6360		98.90%
PDSS	5	37.23	(21.47–56.27)	471	1522		97.50%
SDS	4	28.17	(21.30–36.24)	1231	4248		95.90%
PHQ-2	5	18.47	(14.42–23.34)	14,461	105,902		99.30%
Others	23	14.94	(13.06–17.03)				96.10%
Study quality						0.41	
>8	542	17.52	(16.80–18.27)	163,375	1,184,434		98.80%
<8	29	16.03	(12.98–19.63)	8967	51,931		98.90%
Study period						0.56	
4 weeks–3 months	342	15.35	(14.10–16.70)	55,359	918,858		98.20%
3 months–6 months	89	15.92	(14.03–18.02)	26,031	277,293		99.10%
6 months–12 months	67	17.89	(13.32–23.59)	55,092	1,560,464		99.90%
Longer than 12 months	15	17.95	(13.80–23.01)	1781	11,374		96.60%

Source: [2].

Table 1.
Subgroup analysis for PPD prevalence among women.

various risk factors that are more prevalent in these countries, including intimate partner violence, poverty, childhood abuse, maternal low educational attainment, and lack of social support [3]. The current fertility rate for Australia (a high-income country) in 2021 was 1.794 births per woman [4]. In 2021, there were 309,996 registered births in Australia, and the birth rate was 61 births per 1000 women of reproductive age.

It has been estimated that in Australia, 7 to 15% of pregnant women and 6 to 20% of mothers of infants up to 4 months of age will experience depression [5].

Post-Traumatic Stress Disorder, anxiety and depression may co-occur, with differing exhibiting symptomatology and signs, requiring different treatments [6–8]. Postpartum depression is a form of severe depression after birth that inhibits daily functioning and requires management. It can occur within days, weeks, or months after childbirth and extend beyond the first postpartum year. A woman with postpartum depression may have feelings of anxiety, despair, irritability and sadness to a severe extent [9]. High levels of antenatal (state) anxiety and trait anxiety may be an important predictor of postnatal anxiety and mood disorders, while co-morbidity of depression and anxiety disorders are common [10–14]. Postnatal mood disorders include obsessive compulsive disorder, social phobia, specific phobia, panic disorder and post-traumatic Stress Disorder, generalised anxiety disorder (GAD), and are commonly reported as prevalent as depressive disorders in the postnatal period (Fairbrother et al., 2016, as cited in [15]). The long-term effects of maternal depression include delays in children's cognitive and social development [16]; and emotional and behavioural problems [17–25] and breakdown of relationships [21, 26]; Maternal anxiety and depression may adversely affect the pregnancy, birth and early mother-infant relationships [27].

The postnatal period is a demanding life stage with parental concerns about sleep deprivation, infant health, new additional responsibilities, breastfeeding and birth recovery. Various identified psychosocial risk factors (sleep, education and relationship quality) have been associated with maternal postnatal anxiety symptoms; therefore, there is an opportunity for early identification and intervention from various health professionals [28].

Postnatal psychosocial care promotes enabling women to make the emotional and social adaptations that are necessary for successful functioning as a mother. Any postnatal maternal maternity experience involves some degree of disturbed sleep, bodily changes, anxiety, fatigue, maternal changes, and may also include coping with deteriorations in physical health through various other health changes. Therefore, mental health issues such as anxiety and depression do not exist as silos: other important aspects of psychological well-being such as self-esteem, quality of life, a sense of control, worry, and sleep, birth history, early parenthood experiences with infant feeding have also been independently associated with psychological outcomes for postnatal women, and should be considered equivalently important during the assessment of women's maternal experiences [29].

There is a direct link between postnatal maternal anxiety, stress and depression and poor obstetric and child outcomes. The early identification of women either at risk, or symptomatic of anxiety and depression, facilitates referral for timely and appropriate treatment [19]. There is substantial evidence internationally that all women during the postnatal period should be assessed for postnatal maternal stress, anxiety, and depression and their associated risk factors [6, 15, 30–35]. Next, we explore postnatal mental health screening and assessment in Australia.

1.2 Postnatal mental health screening

1.2.1 The Australian context

The evidence of the benefit of antenatal psychosocial assessment and depression screening has been sufficient to lead the implementation of screening in public hospitals in all states of Australia and scarcely in private hospitals. In Sydney specifically, the SAFE START perinatal mental health policy directive and clinical practice guidelines have been in place in a number of large public maternity hospitals since 2010 [36] with the Integrated Perinatal Care (IPC) model of care implemented in some metropolitan settings. However, since 2010, there have been changes to the SAFESTART policy. SAFESTART has been mandated in all public hospitals in New South Wales, Australia and has been widely accepted and implemented. An Australian Commonwealth Government review and update of the Australian Perinatal Mental Health Guidelines was completed in 2017 and 2023 by the National Centre of Perinatal Excellence (COPE) [15, 37]. These guidelines accentuate the necessity to understand the evidence for screening and to identify and address barriers to implementing psychosocial screening in all healthcare sectors. Actions and procedures by appropriate health professionals are needed to provide solutions and resources for what has been identified by screening postnatal women. Improvements include improved detection of depression, improved treatment and, most importantly, to improved health outcomes [37].

The recommendations of the National Guideline [37] is that women should be provided with universal routine screening for depression postnatally in all Australian hospitals, both private and public [5, 36]. In addition, screening could be incorporated into obstetric shared care offered in general practice by G.P's. However, currently, the extent of implementation of screening in private health services in Australia is unknown. The Australian Institute of Health and Welfare [38] stated that 28% of women who give birth in Australia will choose to do so as private patients in private hospitals, yet little is known about the utilisation of psychosocial screening and assessment in the private sector [39]. In Australia, the main dissimilarity between public and private healthcare are the choice of an admitting obstetrician or doctor, admissions to private rooms, and fees charged for services rendered. Private providers offer various models of obstetric care, and despite Australian National guidelines recommending the implementation of screening in all sectors, it is concerning that standards for perinatal mental health remain chiefly absent from private sector policies and processes [40].

A proportion of women will access health care services in the postnatal period. This is the ideal opportunity for health professionals to identify those at risk of depression, anxiety, or other psychosocial issues, if health professionals are educated to identify risk factors effectively, are confident in questioning women and discussing symptoms, and that an appropriate local referral process is in place. Routine postnatal mental health screening has the capacity to act as a potential preventive strategy for postnatal mental illness in women [8], and is a clear strategy for health promotion and early intervention for the woman, her partner and the infant [6].

Postnatal emotional/mental health disorders are a significant public health issue because of their potential to negatively affect infant attachment security, the maternal-infant relationship, and increase the risk of affective disorders, social behavioural problems, and cognitive delays in young children [19]. Anxiety and depression often remain undetected in childbearing women despite health professionals being available during the postnatal period to identify, prevent, and treat emotional/mental health disturbances [19]. Further, efficient psychosocial care may be affected by service or systematic issues including lack of appropriate training and support, limited staff numbers, and unfamiliarity with screening tools. Within the Australian National Health and Medical Research Council's (NHMRC) Clinical Practice Guidelines for Depression and Related Disorders in the Postnatal Period, universal screening for postnatal depression is anticipated to be completed by relevant health professionals [41]. In private obstetric care, obstetricians are the responsible clinician for ensuring that postnatal psychological screening, assessment, referral and the Edinburgh Postnatal Depression Scale (EPDS) is offered.

Postnatal psychosocial assessment is crucial for the provision of comprehensive clinical care and the development of customised maternal management plans, requiring the clinician to have adequate information with which to make shared clinical decisions/referrals. The universal application and routine use of psychosocial risk and depression assessment/screening has developed as a significant health initiative [42]. Postnatal Psychosocial risk assessment and depression screening can be readily integrated into postnatal care but involves skilled clinical evaluation of the identification of psychological, demographic, social, and physical factors known to affect postnatal mental health for mother and infant, including current distress/depressive symptoms that may be identified in the mother [6, 43]. As important, and underpinning the implementation of universal psychosocial assessment, is the identification of adequate local referral pathways. Appropriate services to address the identified needs of women as experiencing mild or moderate issues, being at risk, or experiencing severe and/or complex mental illness need to be reachable and available to all women identified by assessment or screening. The broad range of services and sectors required for appropriate and timely referral involves developing care that is effectively networked, collaborative and receptive to the involved family [6].

1.2.2 The private sector in Australia

As the prevalence of anxiety or depression and substance use increases in the general population, these issues are likely to become more evident in postnatal care and in both the public and private obstetric settings [44]. Substance use, anxiety and depression can be effectively treated postnatally; however, these conditions are often not identified and therefore remain undertreated. Private obstetricians are often the first, and sometimes the sole provider of healthcare to women and alike primary care providers, have an increasing role in the early detection of postnatal mental health/mood disorders. Although postnatal depression and anxiety are recognised as frequent complications of pregnancy and childbirth, screening and detection of depression by private obstetric prenatal care providers is currently insufficient [44].

Women are not routinely or universally screened postnatally for psychosocial risk factors, depression and anxiety in the private sector in Australia [44]. There are limited studies that explore health professionals' views on screening or perceived barriers to the screening process. In one study, however [10], health professionals were interviewed about their perceptions of psychosocial screening in the private sector. Suggestions were made that appropriate education and training of midwives was needed, that high-risk women needed to be flagged to the midwives, to initiate more in-house resources and external resources/community links and to employ a key midwife with interest and expertise in psychosocial screening. Health professionals interviewed in the private sector identified the benefits of psychosocial screening for women but also the barriers to screening. Midwives had various views on psychosocial screening and assessment in the private sector. Some midwives indicated concern about a woman's postnatal mental health/psychosocial risk factors; however, others expressed apprehension that this was not part of their midwifery role. Some midwives were fearsome of what may be revealed by the woman and how to deal with it. There was an identified concern that obstetricians did not take seriously any concerns highlighted by the midwife about a woman's psychosocial issues when reported to them. There was a sense of a lack of 'ownership' of the women and, therefore, a feeling of powerlessness in addressing their needs. This emphasises the need to educate and support midwives working in the private sector on their important role in enriching the postnatal mental health of women within their direct care. Their role includes capability for prevention, health promotion and early intervention to benefit not only the woman, but her whole family. In response to this, as the developer of the Australian National Guideline, the Centre of Perinatal Excellence [37] provides free, accredited online training for frontline health professionals to support their training needs and ensure confidence, and competence in screening and having the conversation, as well as identifying timely and appropriate postnatal mental health pathways.

Women birthing in the private sector would also benefit from being able to access the array of resources provided in the public sector to support their postnatal mental health care. Collaborative partnerships between public, private and non-government service providers can help support the delivery of appropriate obstetric care and ensure that privately insured women have just access to appropriate mental health care services. As private obstetric providers meet the contemporary challenges of addressing postnatal mental health, there is a substantial demand on the duty of care and capacity of these workforces to undertake universal mental health screening/assessment, to access training programmes, to identify and access relevant referral pathways for and follow-up care, and to ensure organisational and professional policies exist to sustain this process and the staff involved. It is extraordinary that Australian National standards for postnatal mental health are not yet endorsed or incorporated into the private sectors continuous quality improvement processes, including the Australian private hospital accreditation standards. As a result, patient who are paying for a higher level of care are in fact receiving a lower level of care, with respect to emotional and mental health at this vulnerable life stage [44].

However, it is generally established that postnatal screening should not occur without appropriate evidence-based interventions, adequate training and support for staff, and adequate local referral pathways [45]. A vast range of services are required to meet the diverse needs of women identified as being at mild or moderate risk of postnatal depression and or anxiety [6, 46], or experiencing complex or severe mental illness. Referral processes for women with an existing or previous psychiatric disorder also need to be available [47]. An effective model for enhancing communication and continuity between primary and specialist/community-based health services and midwives, is essential to ensure that women who may gain from early intervention and treatment programmes or prevention [42, 48, 49] have 24-hour access to psychiatric or psychological advice and support if they develop symptoms between each obstetric appointments.

In addition to the substantial and still emerging postnatal mental health evidence-base endorsing improved outcomes for mother and infant, these findings support the case for the universal implementation of postnatal screening of depression and anxiety [15, 50], regardless of which health sector a woman chooses to receive obstetric care. The profile of women in the private sector in NSW, Australia is not dissimilar to women choosing to birth in the public sector (**Tables 2** and **3**). It is crucial through screening/assessment, to identify postnatal risk factors and symptoms of anxiety or depression and to provide appropriate support to assist women who need help. However, the identification of women experiencing symptoms and risk factors of anxiety or depression postnatally, implies that resources, education and support will be offered throughout the postnatal period, and that referral to appropriate services and support systems will be offered [42]. Barriers exist for postnatal mental health screening, that must be addressed.

Maternal profile comparisons State-wide (NSW) Midwives Data Collection*	Local regional data (from NSW Midwives Data Collection)	Local public hospital	Study site audit
N = 98,141 n (%) 95% CI	N = 3823 n (%) 95% CI	N = 376 n (%) 95% CI	N = 407 N (%) 95% CI
Age (years) 15–19 3144 (3.2) *3.1–3.3*	169 (4.4) *3.8–5.1*	25 (6.6) *4.5–9.6*	1 (0.2) Not applicable
20–24 12,694 (12.9) *12.7–13.1*	616 (16.1) *15.0–17.3*	81 (21.5) *17.7–26.0*	11 (2.7) 1.5–4.8
25–29 26,769 (27.3) *27.0–27.6*	1128 (29.5) 28.1–31.0	118 (31.4) *26.9–36.2*	106 (26.2) 22.1–30.7
30–34 32,385 (33.0) *32.7–33.3*	1140 (29.8) 28.4–31.3	90 (23.9) *19.9 28.5*	163 (40.2) 35.6–45.1
35–39 18,534 (18.9) *18.6–19.1*	610 (16.0) *14.8–17.2*	43 (11.4) *8.6–15.1*	107 (26.4) 22.4–30.9
40–44 4314 (4.4) *4.3–4.5*	153 (4.0) *3.4–4.7*	18 (4.8) *3.0–7.4*	16 (4.0) 2.4–6.3
> 45 266 (0.3) .2–3	6 (0.2) *.1–.3*	1 (0.3) *Not applicable*	3 (0.7) 0.3–2.2
Born outside Australia 34,342 (35) *34.7–35.3*	252 (6.6) *5.8–7.4*	54 (14.5) *11.2–18.3*	46 (11.4) 8.6–14.8
Primipara[#] 43,140 (44.0) *43.6–44.3*	missing	52 (19.8) *15.5–25.1*	164 (40.5) 35.8–45.3
Multipara[#] 54,985 (56.0) *55.7–56.3*	Missing	210 (80.2) *74.9–84.5*	241 (59.5) 34.7–64.2
Did not smoke during pregnancy 87,580 (89.2) *89.0–89.4*	3398(88.9) *87.8–89.8*	319 (84.8) *80.9–88.1*	407 (100)

Centre for Epidemiology and Evidence. New South Wales Mothers and Babies 2012. Sydney: NSW Ministry of Health, 2014 (Midwives data collected in 2012).[#]Denominator for Local Public Hospital for primipara and multipara n = 262, missing values not included.

Table 2.
Compares local and NSW data.

Variable	Local Public Hospital N = 376 n (%)	Study Site Audit N = 407 n (%)	Significance	Effect size
Age (years)[a] Mean SD	28.3 6.0	32.0 4.4	p < .001	.70[y]
Born outside Australia[c] Yes No	54 (14.5) 322 (85.6)	46 (11.4) 359 (88.6)	$\chi2(1) = 1.7$ p = .194	-.05[z]
Intention to breastfeed[c] Yes No	331 (88.0) 45 (12.0)	400 (98.8) 5 (1.2)	$\chi2(1) = 37.5$ p < .001	-.22[z]
Parity[c] 0 1 2 3 4 Missing[#]	52 (19.8) 111(42.4) 64 (24.4) 28 (10.7) 7 (2.7) 114	164 (40.5) 158 (39.0) 68 (16.8) 11 (1.6) 4 (1.0) 0	$\chi2(4) = 46.1$ p < .001	.26[z]

Variable	Local Public Hospital N = 376 n (%)	Study Site Audit N = 407 n (%)	Significance	Effect size
Attended antenatal classes[c] Yes No	142 (37.8) 234 (62.2)	117 (28.9) 288 (71.1)	χ2(1) = 6.9 p = .008	.094[z]
Non- Smoker[c] Yes No Missing[#]	319 (86.2) 51 (13.8) 6 (1.6)	407 (100) 0 (0) 0 (0)	χ2(1) = 59.7 p < .001	.28[z]
Non-Drinker[c] Yes No Missing[#]	360 (97.0) 11 (3.0) 5 (1.3)	407 (100) 0 (0) 0 (0)	χ2(1) = 12.2 p < .001	.12[z]
History of depression/or anxiety[c] Yes No Missing[#]	116 (31.4) 253 (68.6) 7 (1.3)	59 (14.8) 346 (85.4) 0 (0)	χ2(1) = 30.4 p < .001	.20[z]

[a]*t test.*
[c]*Chi-square test.*
[#]*Missing values not included in the denominator for calculation of proportions of valid data reported in table or Chi-square tests. The proportion Missing is based on the total sample size.*
[y]*d effect size .2 = small, .5 = medium, .8 = large.*
[z]*Phi and Cramer's V effect size .1 = small, .3 = medium, .5 = large.*

Table 3.
Profile of women choosing local public and private obstetric care.

1.3 Barriers to postnatal mental health screening

The evidence of value and need for antenatal psychosocial assessment and depression screening has been abundant to lead to the implementation of screening in public hospitals in all states of Australia. However, details of the implementation of postnatal screening in private obstetric settings is unknown [44]. As any successful implementation depends on the identification of local barriers it is essential to identify actual or perceived barriers that may exist for the implementation of evidence-based postnatal screening interventions in private obstetric care [40]. Women who experience the stressors that are related to an increased risk, or an indication of postnatal mental health disorders should be assessed and offered referral to appropriate services, regardless of their chosen health sector.

1.4 Health care provider barriers

There are identified health care provider barriers to psychosocial screening and assessment. These include patient barriers: stigma, fear, denial. Provider and system barriers; time, a lack of skills, confidence or facilities, managerial support, the authority to implement change and a failure to follow-up referral recommendations. Feelings of discomfort are salient in the literature, in fact, midwives, obstetricians, physicians and paediatricians all report being uncomfortable with screening [40]. While different health professionals (midwives, obstetricians, General Practitioners, paediatricians, health visitors) are interested in the psychosocial well-being of women, and they acknowledge that it is a significant part of their role, screening is not being universally achieved [5]. Although psychosocial and depression screening is mandated in the public sector in Australia, a recent study of 30 Women's Healthcare Australasia (WHA) members found that only 70% were using the EPDS in the antenatal period [5]. Of the 30 members who had implemented antenatal screening, 70% screened for risk of developing depression [5], but only two (20%) used the recommended antenatal risk questionnaire (ANRQ) [5].

1.5 Barriers to antenatal psychosocial assessment and depression screening in private hospital settings

Sources of barriers to the implementation of psychosocial and depression screening in private obstetric settings include barriers for women and their families, Health professional barriers, Organisation or provider barriers [40].

Collaborative postnatal care pathways have been suggested for improving liaison between mental health maternity, and primary care services [51], with a specific point of contact enabling this process by providing specialist information and advice. Therefore, a sustainable model of postnatal mental health care in private obstetrics may involve psychoeducation provided by the midwife at the various clinic appointments and during antenatal classes and a postnatal liaison nurse to screen/assess, support, refer and follow-up women identified as at risk and correspond with women who decline help. Working within a collaborative care model with a postnatal liaison nurse and mental health care providers could guide treatment options to ensure women's support. There is also some evidence that nurse-led counselling, peer support models of care and home visitors may also be effective supports for women [52]. Additionally, the Australian Government initiative "My Health Record" may be able to connect additional information regarding women's health for their various healthcare providers [53].

Women who have private obstetric care have a continuity of care with their obstetrician; however, obstetric appointments are mainly focused on physiological factors associated with the pregnancy rather than psychosocial/mental health factors. Given the known prevalence of antenatal depression, anxiety and other risk factors, it is essential that health care providers view the assessment of mental health as being equally important as the assessment of physical health [13]. The Royal Australian and New Zealand College of Obstetricians and Gynaecologists (RANZCOG) have recommended that all obstetricians screen and assess women for postnatal mental health risks and disorders [54]. Since obstetricians see women consistently during the perinatal period, they are in a prime position to assess, screen and refer women, partially because they have built a rapport with the woman and may notice changes in her circumstances, or psychosocial/mental health risk factors. Although there are identified barriers, there are solutions/recommendations to address these barriers.

2. Solutions/recommendations

2.1 iCOPE

An initiative in Victoria, Australia is currently being used to improve psychosocial screening and assessment uptake in the public sector. iCOPE screening was initially piloted in Victoria and following its positive outcomes has been fully funded to be made available nationally to every public maternity hospital in Australia. Victoria was the first state to take up this state-wide, and in the first year of implementation screening is being digitally implemented across 90 locations and over 20,000 screens conducted across maternity (90% of public hospitals) and postnatal settings (85% MCH settings). In line with best practice [15, 37] the Antenatal Risk Questionnaire/Post Risk Questionnaire

(ANRQ/PNRQ) have been implemented. There has been development of iCOPE Digital psychosocial screening under the Commonwealth's Perinatal Mental Health Check up until July 2025. This includes administration of the Edinburgh Postnatal Depression Scale (EPDS) and the ANQR/PNQR screening tools. This has been initiated in 75% of public hospitals and child and family health services in Victoria. The digital screening tool is available in 25 different languages. As part of the development of the 2023 Guideline, recommendations were given with respect to screening for fathers and partners. Here adaptions were made to the ANRQ/PNRQ and lower cut-off scores applied to the EPDS or use of the K10. These tools and scoring algorithms have been programmed into iCOPE and also digitally available. However, since they are not deemed to be 'the patient' if screening was positive, they would need to access their General Practitioner for follow-up. iCOPE is one example of an initiative in Australia (a high-income country). The digital tool is also available, and is being used within the private sector by OBGYNS. As this is not funded under the Perinatal Mental Health Check Program, access to iCOPE at the expense of the private obstetrician or hospital, however costs can be off-set by Medicare Benefits Schedule (MBS) item number for screening antenatally (16,590/16591 and 16,522) and Postnatally (16407). More information can be found here—https://www.cope.org.au/perinatal-mental-health-check/digital-screening-in-the-private-sector/

2.2 Australian midwifery models of care

Within Australia there are various midwifery models of care including; public hospital care, team midwifery, midwifery group practice case load care and private midwifery care [55]. Midwives may be able to address implementation gaps by providing postnatal psychosocial screening and assessment for women in the private sector, especially since there are financial initiatives via a Medicare rebate for obstetricians for screening. Collaborative obstetric care models that employ midwives with expertise and interest in psychosocial screening as key contacts for postnatal integrated care may offer a successful future solution. The difficulty for midwives working in the private sector is that they often do not have an ongoing relationship with the woman and therefore have a limited opportunity to assess/screen or identify risk factors/disorders [44]. Contributing factors that may influence the approach a midwife takes towards psychosocial screening and assessment include organisational support for continuing education, their experience as a midwife, training and exposure to the practice of others, their own personal life experience, clinical supervision opportunities, and the model of midwifery care within their setting or organisation. Midwives seem willing to have a more substantial role in recommending appropriate psychosocial treatment strategies to women with postnatal depression, however, further training is often required to ensure both confidence and competence in their psychosocial assessment and management of women [10]. Similarly, the majority of obstetricians and/or gynaecologists consider that they have a responsibility to identify depression but may not have the appropriate training and resources to screen for and treat depression. It is also evident that some maternity care providers may be reluctant to ask about depression, and women themselves may be unwilling to disclose their experiences [10, 14].

3. Training and support

Reviews of both the SAFESTART and Beyond Blue guideline implementations indicate that additional training and support are required for primary health care staff, including midwives and child and family health nurses to undertake psychosocial and depression screening and to provide a more psychosocial emphasis in their work. A comprehensive schedule of recommended psychosocial screening and assessment training at basic, intermediate and advanced [37].

A training model must include the further education of as many midwives as possible on psychosocial screening and risk factors, implementing the assessment/screening process, processes for follow-up, and the establishment of referral pathways, with ongoing professional development workshops to support staff attrition. However, this will only be successful if the individual health care service is supportive of the intervention, including making a substantive commitment. The private sector will be required to engage and facilitate interdisciplinary collaboration and interest and make a financial commitment to additional resources (including time) for psychosocial screening within their private model of obstetric care [44].

4. Access to services

Women who chose to give birth in the private sector may also sporadically require access to mental health resources within the public sector to support their care. However, questions regarding private insurance, private providers, and equity of access to community-based public postnatal mental health services have consistently been concluded and not dealt with. The formation of impending collaborative partnerships between public, private, and Non-Government Organisation service providers will be key to appropriately supporting the mental health care of postnatal women who choose to give birth in the private sector. In order to access equitable and adequate postnatal mental health care, Australian women must be able to transfer straightforwardly between a broad range of services and sectors [44].

Key mental health partner organisations working with the private sector (such as St John of God Health Care) express the possibilities for collaborative partnerships to promote the wider implementation of mental health care plans between private settings. While concern for personal privacy is undoubtedly important, the introduction of electronic health records across Australia further increases opportunities for discussion on the appropriate and timely sharing of health information. Similarly, the upholding of collaborative practices and partnerships will be crucial for ongoing and sustained change. COPE has developed a national perinatal mental health directory of services to support timely and accurate referral that is funded by the Commonwealth Government [37].

5. Workforce

As the Australian private health sector continues to expand, service accountability for identifying and supporting postnatal mental health care will continue to challenge the capacity of these organisations to ensure their workforces are maintained to undertake routine universal postnatal screening and assessment [5, 15]. Australian National standards for perinatal mental health have already been developed and endorsed [6, 15, 37, 45, 46] and currently need to be introduced into the continuous quality improvement processes of private sector facilities in order to meet the Australian hospital accreditation requirements. In addition, private sector providers must increase staff access to continuous professional education/development programmes, to find relevant pathways to collaborative care and ensure that professional and organisational policies and procedures are developed to support this ongoing process [6, 15, 45, 46].

While privately funded obstetric services providers are recommended to encompass the recommendations of the National Guidelines [37] for universal postnatal screening, it appears that application has been widely lacking. The most recent National Perinatal Mental Health Guideline from the Centre of Perinatal Excellence (COPE) [37] has now superseded the initial Beyond Blue Guidelines that were developed and endorsed by NHMRC [6, 45, 46] and this new guideline recommends that ALL hospitals screen and assess women for postnatal mental health risk factors and issues including private obstetric providers. The postnatal period offers an opportunistic time for prevention, promotion, identification, and early intervention of women's mental health. However, there have been inequitable opportunities to support women postnatally within existing systems in training, assessment and referral pathways to continuing care, other than iCOPE training since 2013 [5, 15]. Future private provider services that implement the National Perinatal Health Guideline will necessitate enhanced engagement with specialist postnatal mental health services and also community healthcare and primary healthcare services for sustaining fundamental approaches, functions and activities.

6. Health sector regulations

The private sector is not governed by the same regulations, governance or policies of the Australian Government public sector. Local level decisions are made within each individual hospital, Board of Directors or company electing to prioritise a woman's psychosocial well-being through risk assessment, management and referral. Nonetheless, as stated by Gemmill [56], electing not to perform postnatal screening and assessment due to a lack of mental health resources, or the perception that it is too complex, is discounting the surmountable evidence-based international literature on the pertinent role of psychosocial well-being on maternal and infant outcomes. The administration of a postnatal screening assessment that identifies women at risk of postnatal anxiety and depression/currently experiencing anxiety/depression should be considered best (evidence-based) practice in order to support the long-term well-being of mother and baby [6, 15, 45, 46, 57].

Within private obstetric care, obstetricians are the answerable health professional for ensuring that psychosocial assessment and screening with the EPDS is utilised. Relevant health care providers, including midwives at the hospital at which the woman will give birth, need to be informed if there are concerns and relevant information consistently and clearly documented in the women's notes and discharge summary [15].

It is clearly recommended that existing state-wide midwifery databases be made able to link private and public hospital data with community or General Practitioner services across Australia to identify women at risk of/with postnatal mental health problems [6, 45, 46]. The federal government's introduction of an electronic health record may be useful, contributing to improved data sharing and linkage between service providers. iCOPE is also integrated with My Health Record in Australia.

7. Solutions/recommendations conclusion

In conclusion, a sustainable model of postnatal mental health care in private obstetrics might include screening, assessment referral and psychoeducation provided by a midwife. Alternatively, a committed postnatal liaison nurse (midwife) to screen, refer, support and follow up women identified as at risk/concern and also engage with women who decline help. The role of the midwife could be advanced further to provide improved continuity in relation to screening and support for mental health. This could be through the development of a role for Advanced Midwifery Practitioners, who are named and regulated as specialised mental health midwives. This could additionally be endorsed by specialist postgraduate or other higher education programmes for both midwives and obstetricians. There are also online training and face to face training programmes available for midwives – on perinatal screening and assessment. These include the COPE Basic Skills in Perinatal Mental Health, KMMS module for screening Australian First Nations (now also part of iCOPE) women and perinatal loss in practice. The perinatal loss in practice is a practical, comprehensive course for Therapists, including Psychologists, Psychiatrists, Social Workers, Counsellors, and Mental Health Nurses, who work with clients who have experienced miscarriage, stillbirth, and newborn loss.

More experienced midwives and child and family health nurses [58] are known to utilise a variety of strategies to make clinical decisions and to utilise critical thinking to detect women who require follow-up support for postnatal mental health disorders [59]. Midwives who have more experience in psychosocial screening and assessment and who have developed effective screening and problem-solving abilities are in the idyllic position to mentor and support less experienced midwives, however, it is uncertain whether this peer-mentoring occurs.

More support markedly required to identify and promote family and community-centred approaches to mental well-being for postnatal women, and all Australian families would gain from improved information regarding the benefits, purpose and aims of postnatal mental health screening and assessment. A wide-based educational communication strategy is advised to enhance awareness of postnatal mental health issues, particularly the impact on infant well-being and development and the needs of the family unit. A simultaneous consultation strategy is necessary to identify additional tactics to engage key stakeholders, including private obstetric service providers, in the implementation and evaluation of this essential health promotion campaign. In addition, universal routine psychosocial screening/assessment should be conducted postnatally, regardless of the outcome of antenatal screening.

The Centre of Perinatal Excellence (COPE) has developed an e-directory to assist women in finding local support for emotional and mental health problems perinatally. It includes over 700 services. This includes services and professionals that have a special focus on emotional and mental health during pregnancy and following the birth of a baby. This directory could be promoted to postnatal women by health care professionals. There is also a preparation for parenthood psychoeducation programme through COPE for women. In addition, there is a free ready-to-cope psychoeducation app available for women called, 'Ready to Cope'. This provides weekly updates for pregnant woman, men and non-birthing partners until the completion of their first year of parenting. Monash University have also demonstrated that iCOPE can be successfully used with refugee women by offering screening in their own language [60].

8. Conclusion

In conclusion, postnatal mental health is clearly a contemporary challenge as the risks associated with this have long-term effects on the mother, infant and their family. Projected costs for not treating depression and anxiety in 2013 were estimated to be $538 million during the perinatal period; however, detection and early intervention can reduce costs. Appropriate and timely psychosocial screening and assessment in the postnatal period is essential for postnatal women, their families, and outcomes. However, there are identified barriers to psychosocial assessment and screening globally – many of which have now been rectified through the development and application of innovative digital solutions to psychoeducation, screening referral and health professional training. These barriers need to be identified and addressed locally. Health care professionals are responsible for psychosocial screening and assessment of postnatal women. This contemporary challenge needs to be addressed urgently.

Author details

Tanya Connell
The University of Sydney, Australia

*Address all correspondence to: tanya_connell@bigpond.com

IntechOpen

© 2023 The Author(s). Licensee IntechOpen. This chapter is distributed under the terms of the Creative Commons Attribution License (http://creativecommons.org/licenses/by/3.0), which permits unrestricted use, distribution, and reproduction in any medium, provided the original work is properly cited.

References

[1] Phua DY, Kee MKZL, Koh DXP, Rifkin-Graboi A, Daniels M, Chen H, et al. Positive maternal mental health during pregnancy associated with specific forms of adaptive development in early childhood: Evidence from a longitudinal study. Development and Psychopathology. 2017;**29**(5):1573-1587. DOI: 10.1017/S0954579417001249. Erratum in: Dev Psychopathol. 2018 Oct;30(4):1547

[2] Wang Z, Jiaye L, Huan S, Cai ZF, Xia LY, Xiong X, et al. Mapping global prevalence of depression among postpartum women. Translational. Psychiatry. 2021;**11**:543

[3] Fatori D, Fonseca ZP, Polanczyk GV. A global challenge: Maternal depression and offspring mental disorders. European Child & Adolescent Psychiatry. 2020;**29**:569-571

[4] Australian Bureau of Statistics. Births. Australia: ABS; 2021. Available from: https://www.abs.gov.au/statistics/people/population/births-australia/latest-release

[5] Fisher J, Chatham C, Haseler S, McGaw B, Thompson J. Uneven implementation of the National Perinatal Depression Initiative: Findings from a survey of Australian women's hospitals. Australian & New Zealand Journal of Obstetrics & Gynaecology. 2012;**52**(6):559-564

[6] Beyond Blue. Beyond Blue Perinatal Mental Health National Action Plan, 2008-2011. Beyond Blue; 2008. Available from: www.beyondblue.org.au/docs/default-source/8.-perinatal-documents/bw0125-report-beyondblues-perinatal-mental-health-(nap)-full-report.pdf?sfvrsn=2

[7] Martin CR. Perinatal Mental Health: A Clinical Guide. UK: British Library Catalogue in Publication Data; 2012. M&K Update. Kindle Edition

[8] Priest SR, Austin M, Barnett BB, Buist A. A psychosocial risk assessment model (PRAM) for use with pregnant and postpartum women in primary care settings. Archives of Women's Mental Health. 2008;**11**(5-6):307-317

[9] MedicineNet. Post Partum Depression. MedicineNet; 2019. Available from: https://www.medicinenet.com/script/main/art.asp?articlekey=151667

[10] Connell T. Perinatal psychosocial assessment-what are the views of health professionals working in the private obstetric sector? Journal of Women's Health and Development. 2019;**2**(4):112-118

[11] Connell T. Pre and postnatal anxiety in women delivering in a private obstetric hospital. Journal of Women's Health and Development. 2019;**2**:1116-1119

[12] Connell T. What are the essential referral pathways for perinatal women? Journal of Women's Health and Development. 2019;**2**(1):001-005

[13] Connell T. What is the health Professional's role in perinatal psychosocial screening assessment and referral in the private sector? Journal of Women's Health and Development. 2019;**2**:1117-11JJ

[14] Connell T. Antenatal psychosocial assessment and depression screening: What are the views of women delivering in the private sector? Journal of Womens Health and Gynecology. 2019;**6**:1-6

[15] Austin MP, Highet N, Expert Working Group. Mental Health Care in the Perinatal Period: Australian Clinical Practice Guideline. Melbourne, VIC: Centre of Perinatal Excellence; 2017. Available from: https://cope.org.au/wp-content/uploads/2017/10/Final-COPE-Perinatal-Mental-Health-Guideline.pdf

[16] Hayes BA, Muller R, Bradley BS. Perinatal depression: A randomized controlled trial of an antenatal education intervention for primiparas. Birth. 2001;**28**(1):28-35

[17] Deave T. Research nurse or nurse researcher: How much value is placed on research undertaken by nurses. Journal of Research in Nursing. 2005;**10**(6):649-657

[18] Deave T, Johnson D. The transition to parenthood: What does it mean for fathers? Journal of Advanced Nursing. 2008;**63**(6):626-633

[19] Glover V. Maternal depression, anxiety and stress during pregnancy and child outcome; what needs to be done. Best Practice & Research in Clinical Obstetrics & Gynaecology. 2014;**28**(1):25-35

[20] Grace SL, Evindar A, Stewart DE. The effect of postpartum depression on child cognitive development and behavior: A review and critical analysis of the literature. Archives of Women's Mental Health. 2003;**6**(4):263-274

[21] Murray L, Cooper P, Stein A. Postnatal depression and infant development. BMJ. 1991;**302**:978-979. DOI: 10.1136/bmj.302.6783.978

[22] O'Connor TG, Heron J, Glover V, Avon Longitudinal Study of Parents and Children Study Team. Antenatal anxiety predicts child behavioral/emotional problems independently of postnatal depression. Journal of the American Academy of Child & Adolescent Psychiatry. 2002;**41**(12):1470-1477

[23] Oates MR. Adverse effects of maternal antenatal anxiety on children: Causal effect or developmental continuum? British Journal of Psychiatry. 2002;**180**:478-479

[24] Rubertsson C et al. Depressive mood in early pregnancy: Prevalence and women at risk in a national Swedish sample. Journal of Reproductive & Infant Psychology. 2003;**21**(2):113-123

[25] Talge NM, Neal C, Glover V. Antenatal maternal stress and long-term effects on child neurodevelopment: How and why? Early stress, translational research and prevention science network fetal and neonatal experience on child and adolescent mental health. Journal of Child Psychology & Psychiatry & Allied Disciplines. 2007;**48**(3-4):245-261

[26] Boath E, Cox J, Lewis M, Jones P, Pryce A. When the cradle falls: The treatment of postnatal depression in a psychiatric day hospital compared with routine primary care. Journal of Affective Disorders. 1999;**53**(2):143-151

[27] Silverman ME, Loudon H. Antenatal reports of pre-pregnancy abuse are associated with symptoms of depression in the postpartum period. Archives of Women's Mental Health. 2010;**13**(9):411-415

[28] Seymour M, Giallo R, Cooklin A, Dunning M. Maternal anxiety, risk factors and parenting in the first post-natal year. Child: Care, Health & Development. 2015;**41**(2):314-323

[29] Jomeen J, Martin CR. The impact of choice of maternity care on psychological health outcomes for women during pregnancy and the postnatal period.

Journal of Clinical Evaluation. 2008;**14**(3):391-398

[30] American Psychiatric Association. The management of depression during pregnancy: A report from the American Psychiatric, Association and the American College of Obstetricians and Gynecologists. Obstetrics & Gynecology. 2009;**114**(3):703-713

[31] Committee on Obstetric Practice. The American College of Obstetricians and Gynecologists Committee opinion no. 630. Screening for perinatal depression. Obstetrics & Gynecology. 2015;**125**(5):1268-1271

[32] National Institute of Care Excellence. NICE guideline supports normal birth. Practising Midwife. 2007;**10**(10):6

[33] National Institute for Health and Care Excellence. Antenatal and Postnatal Mental Health: Clinical Management and Service Guidance. National Institute for Health and Care Excellence; 2014. Available from: https://www.nice.org.uk/guidance/cg192/chapter/1-Recommendations#recognisingmental-health-problems-in-pregnancy-and-the-postnatal-period-and-referral-2

[34] US Preventive Services Taskforce. Screening for depression in adults: US preventive services taskforce recommendation statement. Annals of Internal Medicine. 2009;**151**(11):784-792

[35] US Preventive Services Taskforce. Final Recommendation Statement, Depression in Adults: Screening. 2016. Available from: http://www.uspreventiveservicestaskforce.org/Page/Document/RecommendationStatement

[36] New South Wales Department of Health. NSW Supporting Families Early Package–SAFE START Guidelines: Improving Mental Health Outcomes for Parents and Infants. NSW Department of Health; 2009. Available from: https://www1.health.nsw.gov.au/pds/Active PDS Documents/GL2010_004.pdf

[37] Highet NJ, The Expert Working Group and Expert Subcommittees. Mental Health Care in the Perinatal Period: Australian Clinical Practice Guideline. Melbourne: Centre of Perinatal Excellence (COPE); 2023

[38] Australian Institute of Health & Welfare. Australia's Health 2016. Canberra: AIHW, ACT; 2016

[39] Christl B, Reilly N, Smith M, Sims D, Chavasse F, Austin M-PV. The mental health of mothers of unsettled infants: Is there value in routine psychosocial assessment in this context? Archives of Women's Mental Health. 2013;**16**:391-399

[40] Connell T, Barnett B, Waters D. Barriers to antenatal psychosocial assessment and depression screening in private hospital settings. Women and Birth. 2017;**31**(4):292-298

[41] Jones CJ, Creedy DK, Gamble JA. Australian midwives' awareness and management of antenatal and postpartum depression. Women & Birth. 2012;**25**(1):23-28

[42] Barnett B, Glossop P, Matthey S, Stewart H. Screening in the Context of Integrated Perinatal Care. London. UK: Jessica Kingsley; 2005

[43] Council of Australian Governments. National Action Plan on Mental Health. Council of Australian Governments; 2006. Available from: http://www.coag.gov.au/coag_meeting_outcomes/2006-07-14/docs/nap_mental_health.pdf

[44] Connell T. Psychosocial assessment and depression screening in private

obstetric care [thesis]. Australia: The University of Sydney. Faculty of Medicine and Health, Sydney Nursing School; 2018. Available from: http://hdl.handle.net/2123/20828

[45] Beyond Blue. Annual Report 2009-2010. The National Perinatal Depression Initiative. Beyond Blue; 2010. Available from: http://resources.beyondblue.org.au/prism/file?token=BL/0879

[46] Beyond Blue. The National Depressive Initiative Mental Health National Action Plan 2008-2010 Full Report. Beyond Blue; 2008. Available from: https://www.beyond193blue.org.au/docs/default-source/8.-perinatal-documents/bw0125-report-beyondblues-perinatal-mental-health-(nap)-full-report.pdf?sfvrsn=2

[47] Sidebotham M. Antenatal issues. NICE guideline: Antenatal care under the microscope. British Journal of Midwifery. 2004;**12**(3):137-140

[48] Austin MP, Priest SR. Clinical issues in perinatal mental health: New developments in the detection and treatment of perinatal mood and anxiety disorders. Acta Psychiatrica Scandinavica. 2005;**112**(2):97-104

[49] Buist A, Hayes B, Milgrom J, Barnett B. Not all questions can be answered. Australian & New Zealand Journal of Public Health. 2007;**31**(3):288

[50] Eastwood JG, Phung H, Barnett B. Postnatal depression and socio-demographic risk: Factors associated with Edinburgh depression scale scores in a metropolitan area of New South Wales, Australia. Australian & New Zealand Journal of Psychiatry. 2011;**45**(12):1040-1046. DOI: 10.3109/00048674.2011.619160

[51] Rothera I, Oates M. Managing perinatal mental health: A survey of practitioners' views. British Journal of Midwifery. 2011;**19**(5):304

[52] Milgrom J, Gemmill AW. Identifying Perinatal Depression and Anxiety: Evidence-Based Practice in Screening. Psychosocial Assessment and Management. 1st ed. Chichester, UK: John Wiley & Sons; 2015

[53] Australian Government. My Health Records. Australian Government; n.d. Available from: https://www.myhealthrecord.gov.au/

[54] Royal Australian and New Zealand College of Obstetricians and Gynaecologists. Perinatal Anxiety and Depression. 2015. Available from: https://www.ranzcog.edu.au/Statements-Guidelines

[55] Australian Institute of Health and Welfare. Maternity Models of Care in Australia. AIHW, Australian Government; 2022 [Accessed: July 26, 2022]

[56] Gemmill AW. The long gestation of screening programmes for perinatal depressive disorders. Journal of Psychosomatic Research. 2014;**77**(3):242-243

[57] Pawlby S, Hay DF, Sharp D, Waters CS, O'Keane V. Antenatal depression predicts depression in adolescent offspring: Prospective longitudinal community-based study. Journal of Affective Disorders. 2009;**113**(3):236-243

[58] Rollans M, Schmied V, Kemp L, Meade T. Digging over that old ground: An Australian perspective of women's experience of psychosocial assessment and depression screening in pregnancy and following birth. BMC Women's Health. 2013;**13**:18

[59] Rollans M, Schmied V, Kemp L, Meade T. Negotiating policy into practice: Child and family health nurses' approach to the process of postnatal psychosocial assessment. BMC Health Services Research. 2013;**13**:133

[60] Boyle JA, Willey S, Blackmore R, East C, McBride J, Gray K, et al. Improving mental health in pregnancy for refugee women: Protocol for the implementation and evaluation of a screening program in Melbourne, Australia. JMIR Research Protocols. 2019;**8**(8):e13271. DOI: 10.2196/13271

Chapter 2

Barriers and Challenges in the Acceptance and Continuation of Postpartum Intrauterine Contraceptive Device

Tripti Sinha

Abstract

Postpartum family planning (PPFP) interventions have immense potential to address the unmet contraceptive need in women from the time their baby is delivered till a variable period in their reproductive span. Postpartum intrauterine contraceptive device (PPIUCD) is one among the birth-spacing and birth-limiting contraceptive options. They have most attributes of an ideal contraceptive providing prolonged contraception akin to permanent contraceptives with scope of reversibility should the reproductive intentions of the couple change in future. This appeals to the societies and religious communities, who oppose permanent contraception. However, the acceptance and long-term continuation of the IUCD remains limited to and fails to total fertility rates (TFR) in populations who need it most. Global studies indicate this is often due to service providers' adverse negative perception of PPIUCD, poor counseling skills, lack of technical skills in its insertion, and logistical limitations in various health facilities where deliveries occur, as well as the women's and their family's perspective about it rather than any intrinsic adverse characteristic of the device. The chapter is discourse about PPIUCD from multiple dimensions to define the barriers and challenges to its use in current practice. Interventions suggested may be incorporated into the national PPFP policy and program implementation as it is rolled out as a sustainable population control measure with far-reaching implications.

Keywords: FP, IUCD, PPIUCD, PPFP, counselors, service providers, LMIC, expulsion, missing threads

1. Introduction

The postpartum period in the lives of women in the reproductive age group is characterized by certain features, which are related to her future reproductive performance. She is vulnerable to the risk of an unintended pregnancy (!! surprise/? shock pregnancy), especially in the first year postpartum. This is because she has the common misconception that as long as she breastfeeds her infant, she cannot get pregnant. She is unaware that factors such as the duration and frequency of breastfeeding and any supplementary top-up feeds she may be giving to her child affect the time when ovulation may be resumed postpartum. Such factors account for the unpredictability of the resumption of ovulation and menstruation [1]. Coupled with this is the fact that most couples resume coital relations within a month of delivery [2]. The combined impact of these factors is that the woman is exposed to the risk of a subsequent pregnancy before the optimal delivery-conception interval, thus shortening the inter-delivery interval as well. Such closely -spaced pregnancies are contrary to the recommendations of the World Health Organization (WHO) regarding birth spacing [3]. Data from India show a huge unmet need of contraception as high as 65% in the first postpartum year (USAID India, 2009). Similarly, National Family Health Survey (NFHS), 2005–2006 also showed similar findings in relation to postpartum contraceptive usage as a result of which 65% births occur within 36 months of the previous birth. Similar situation is present in countries such as Pakistan [4, 5].

2. Health, economic, and other societal impact of unmet need for contraception

Postpartum family planning (PPFP) contraceptive options are an effective strategy to reduce this unmet need for contraception [3]. This has the potential to have short-term and long-term impacts on the total fertility rate (TFR) of populations, as well as their maternal, neonatal, and infant morbidity and mortality statistics [6].

PPFP reduces not only the family size but also the number of women seeking induced abortion. However, due to gaping lacunae in PPFP service delivery in LMIC women often suffer from morbidity and mortality related to complications of induced abortion. Women who conceive very soon after childbirth often become aware of their current pregnancy in the late first trimester, or even in the second trimester when she notices a lump in her lower abdomen. She may even have perceived fetal movements. If she has lactational amenorrhea missed periods will not indicate to her that she may be pregnant. If she does not want to continue such late-diagnosed pregnancy the termination itself becomes a protracted and unsafe procedure. Very often such women in their desperation turn to unqualified untrained persons to terminate their pregnancy often in suboptimal settings and beyond the safe limits of pregnancy termination.

If such women who are often multiparous die during the termination they leave behind young children whose care and upbringing are affected having disastrous consequences for their families and the society at large.

3. Status of copper IUCDS as a contraceptive option

The copper-containing intrauterine contraceptive device (Cu T IUCD) in its various designs has been available globally both in the government sector and in private health facilities for several decades. In government facilities, the IUCD is provided free of cost. In private facilities, social marketing strategies often make it available at very subsidized rate so that it becomes affordable for the user. However, the timing of its insertion was restricted to the interval period (i.e. between pregnancies and interval insertion) or immediately following pregnancy termination (post MTP insertion). Apart from registered medical practitioners and specialist obstetricians and gynecologists, nurses and auxiliary nurse midwives trained in insertion procedures were delegated the task of interval IUCD insertions as part of task shifting / sharing approach in the health service delivery system. However, this timing and strategy of contraceptive provision failed to cater to the unmet contraceptive needs of the vulnerable postpartum women. An unintended pregnancy for such women poses risks for their own health as well as that of their children [7–9].

Technical experts on reproductive health and contraception reached the consensus that health care providers (HCP) had the opportunity for IUCD insertion in the immediate postpartum period when the parturient/puerpera was still within a healthcare facility. The delivery site could function both as an institutional delivery setup and contraceptive provision center. Since the commencement of this millennium, this strategy has been rolled out in several low- and middle-income countries (LMIC)—first as pilot projects in a few targeted centers with high delivery rates and then introduced into health facilities at various tiers of health care delivery system [10].

The FIGO initiative is the largest intervention study to date which examined the feasibility and efficacy of PPIUCD as a contraceptive option provided in the basket of choices offered in government hospitals in six LMICs in Asia—India, Nepal, Bangladesh, Sri Lanka, Tanzania, and Kenya [11–15]. The study highlighted certain important observations related not only to the satisfactory rating of the PPIUCD as an effective contraceptive option for women having institutional delivery but also how task-sharing by specialist obstetricians, general duty medical officers trained in vaginal delivery, and staff nurses, and midwives could dramatically increase the number of women who could avail the benefits of the IUCD and leave the health care facility with a highly effective and safe contraceptive option in place in order to protect them from unintended pregnancies. Community health workers like dedicated family planning counselors and ASHAs (accredited social health activists) in India who are oriented and trained in contraceptive counseling can effectively contribute to demand generation in the community for PPIUCD acceptance and continuation.

4. Status of PPIUCD as a viable popular contraceptive option.

PPIUCD has an established reputation as an efficient, safe, reversible, long-acting nonhormonal contraceptive. It is also cost-effective and readily available, with a short learning curve for service providers to learn its insertion technique [16–19]

Despite the promising results elicited by the FIGO endeavor and government enthusiasm and support in the participating six countries, PPIUCD remains an under-utilized contraceptive option and falls short of expectations in lowering fertility rates in those populations, where it is most needed. A recent systemic review on the utilization of PPIUCD globally comes to the conclusion that despite its safety and efficacy it remains an underused contraceptive option [20]. It concludes with the observation that future research is warranted and vital to explore the reasons behind these discouraging trends and the low acceptance and provision of PPIUCDs currently. The analysis needs to be in various dimensions including the innate characteristics of the device and the logistics of its availability and utilization by the service providers. Without an in-depth analysis, it would not be prudent for governments to withdraw it as a freely available, free-of-cost/subsidized option in the contraceptive basket provided by government and private health care setups.

5. Factors affecting contraceptive usage

Various studies have shown that the acceptance and continuation of any contraceptive method is directly related to the efficacy of method counseling, availability and cost of the method, and quality of the involved service delivery system. Given the rigorous quality assurance standards to which Cu-T devices were subjected before being launched as a globally highly-rated contraceptive method, it is imperative to critically examine the service delivery systems in place in various countries. These logistics may be the actual determining/influencing factors affecting the uptake and continuation of PPIUCD in LMIC [21].

6. Women's expectations from a contraceptive method

After having experienced a pregnancy and birthing experience—either vaginal or abdominal—most women would personally prefer to defer any subsequent pregnancy. Whether she can avail of any contraceptive method or not is another issue, which contributes to the proportion of women who have an unmet need for contraception in the postpartum and subsequent period when she resumes coital relations. During this phase of her life, the expectations of women from any contraception, which she would like to use include the following:

Success rate	At par with oral contraceptives, injectables, sterilization
Ectopic pregnancy	<1 per 1000 years of use
Reversal of fertility	Immediately on removal of device
Effect on lactation	None
Need for follow-up visits	Initially after a month at regular postnatal visit, then annually till effective period of contraception lasts when woman can have repeat insertion if desired
Post-insertion abdominal/ pelvic pain or discomfort	Co-exists with after-pains of delivery and woman not unduly concerned
Heavy/irregular vaginal bleeds	Lactation delays menstruation; if periods later bothersome most women respond to conservative management like tranexamic acid and hematinics
Acceptability in communities who eschew permanent contraception	High
Shelf life	Long (5–10 years)
Learning curve for service providers	Short
Cost- effectiveness	High
Instruments needed for insertion	Cheap, minimum number, readily available, reusable, easily sterilized
Anesthesia at vaginal insertions	None
Removal	Usually easy, in OPD, without anesthesia

Table 1.
Positive attributes of PPIUCD as a contraceptive.

1. Protect her against any unwanted and/or mistimed pregnancy

2. Maintain her normal menstrual cycle and flow pattern

3. Not have any effect on her lactation

4. Cause no/minimal side effects

5. Not have any serious adverse effects for her general health

6. Not adversely affect any co-morbidities she may be having concomitantly or their management (**Table 1**).

7. Attributes of an ideal contraceptive

Historically, and even up to current times, the search for an ideal contraceptive method/device continues and remains incomplete and unsuccessful—a single method, which would be acceptable to all women who need and desire contraception globally in developed and developing countries across the board. Given the expectations of the users (male and female clients), service providers, government, and private agencies involved in the logistics and financial aspects of contraception provision, as well as other stakeholders; any contraceptive method should have the following attributes to qualify for the epithet of an ideal contraceptive method:

1. Success rate approaching 100%

2. Minimal chances of ectopic pregnancy in the event of contraceptive failure

3. Minimal or no change from normal menstrual cycle or flow pattern

4. Not have any bothersome side effects disrupting her usual life pattern

5. Not have life-threatening or serious morbid risks for any other systems

6. Not have any adverse impact on any concurrent morbidities she may be suffering from or affect its management

7. Convenient to use for the client

8. Not affect her fertility in the future with easy quick return to fertility on stoppage of use

9. Minimal difference between the success rate for perfect use and typical use

10. Be available either free or at subsidized rates by social marketing

11. Be readily available at government setups and retail over-the-counter outlets

12. Should not place an economic burden on the health services of the government at the expense of other services to be provided by the government also as part of its national health policy

13. Counseling and usage skills are easy to learn by the service providers and support staff involved in contraceptive counseling

14. Long shelf life to reduce wastage of contraceptive resources

15. Should not interfere with normal sexual drive and couple sexual relation [22]

Given these varied aspects of contraceptive usage and provision coupled with the fact that the contraceptive needs and choices of males and females are not constant throughout their reproductive phase of life the search for the single "ideal contraceptive" for all women remains elusive akin to a mirage. It is more reasonable, practical, and feasible to tailor and customize the chosen contraceptive to the dynamics of the user's needs, health, and financial status. The PPIUCD to a large extent provides these benefits [23].

8. Who medical eligibility criteria and PPIUCD

The WHO medical eligibility criteria guideline is a useful clinical tool for contraceptive service providers and counselors. It is available as easy to use "wheel," which should be provided in the contraceptive basket of choices discussed with the clients, whenever they make their contraceptive decisions and choices (**Figure 1a** and **b**).

Against this backdrop, the PPIUCD measures high as a suitable contraceptive for a large section of women for a long period of their life. The following attributes of the PPIUCD have the potential to make it a popular choice for women starting from the immediate postpartum/post abortal/post MTP period to a variable period in months or years depending on the circumstances of the user (**Table 1**).

9. Barriers to acceptance of PIUCD

Despite so many positive attributes of an ideal contraceptive, the PPIUCD has not lived up to the expectations of family planning proponents and those who frame health policies and programs. PPIUCD has not gained the expected widespread acceptance and popularity to have a forceful impact on the fertility indices of most countries, which are hard-pressed to rein in their booming population growth. The reasons contributing to this "below expected" performance need to be examined both by the service providers at the individual and institutional level, as well as the policy makers and funding agencies, which have invested in PPFP and PPIUCD programs in various countries. In most LMICs, use of IUCDs remains extremely low often below 1% [24, 25].

It is a sobering and undeniable fact that the attitude and enthusiasm of any intervention or procedure are directly related to its frequency and appropriateness of use. The author has direct experience of how lack of enthusiasm and unstructured protocol for counseling and provision of PPIUCD in a tertiary care center for institutional deliveries caused the PPIUCD program to nosedive to no insertions after vaginal deliveries and skewed insertions at cesarean sections depending on the enthusiasm

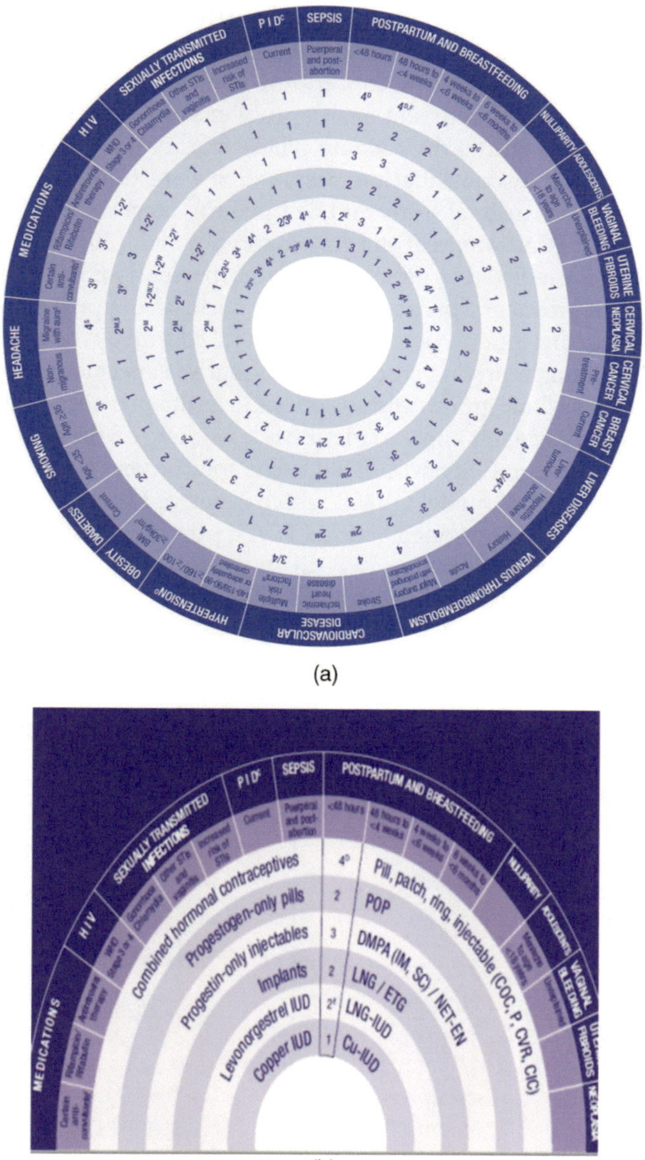

(a)

(b)

Figure 1.
(a) WHO medical eligibility wheel for contraceptives (front) (b) WHO medical eligibility wheel for contraceptives (back).

and motivation of the surgeon performing the cesarean section toward PPIUCD as an effective and safe contraceptive method rather than as indicated by the individual patient's circumstances and needs (unpublished data).

Several studies have examined the perceptions of service providers and allied health workers, as well as users' perceptions about PPIUCD as a contraceptive option. A study by Singh et al. in Bihar, an economically less developed state of Eastern India with high total fertility rate, concluded that the major barriers for acceptance of PPIUCD by the section of the population who were eligible to use it were lack of awareness about PPIUCD, preference for another method vis-a-vis PPIUCD based on personal experience or on shared experience of friends and family users who influenced their choice, husband or family members' disapproval, social or religious taboos, rumors, fears, myths and misconceptions(cancers, migration of PPIUCD to other body organs), past or current health problems or fear of side effects due to a foreign body lodged within their womb. These factors also contributed to the significant removal and discontinuation rates, which were as high as 25.9% in the above-mentioned observational study and damped the success rate of PPIUCD as a game-changer in PPFP initiatives of the government overall [26].

The PPFP index is predicted by descriptive norms, perceptions of the larger community's approval or disapproval of a particular method, normative expectations, rejection of PPFP myths and misconceptions, perceived behavioral control by the user, self-efficacy, and autonomy in making reproductive choices. Normative expectations regarding PPFP intentions vary across ethnic groups and societies. Governments need to acknowledge these sociological determinants and variations while working on the policy and program evolution strategy by integrating norm-based and empowerment strategies [27].

The integrated behavior model (IBM), which is derived from theory of personal belief (TPB) and theory of reasoned action (TRA), provides a valid framework for developing PPFP programs including PPIUCD protocols (**Figure 2**) [27]. It delineates the socioeconomic influences and demographic variables that operate through an individual and their family to shape/define their behavioral intentions collectively. A study from Nigeria reinforced such premises in relation to the PPIUCD. Generally,

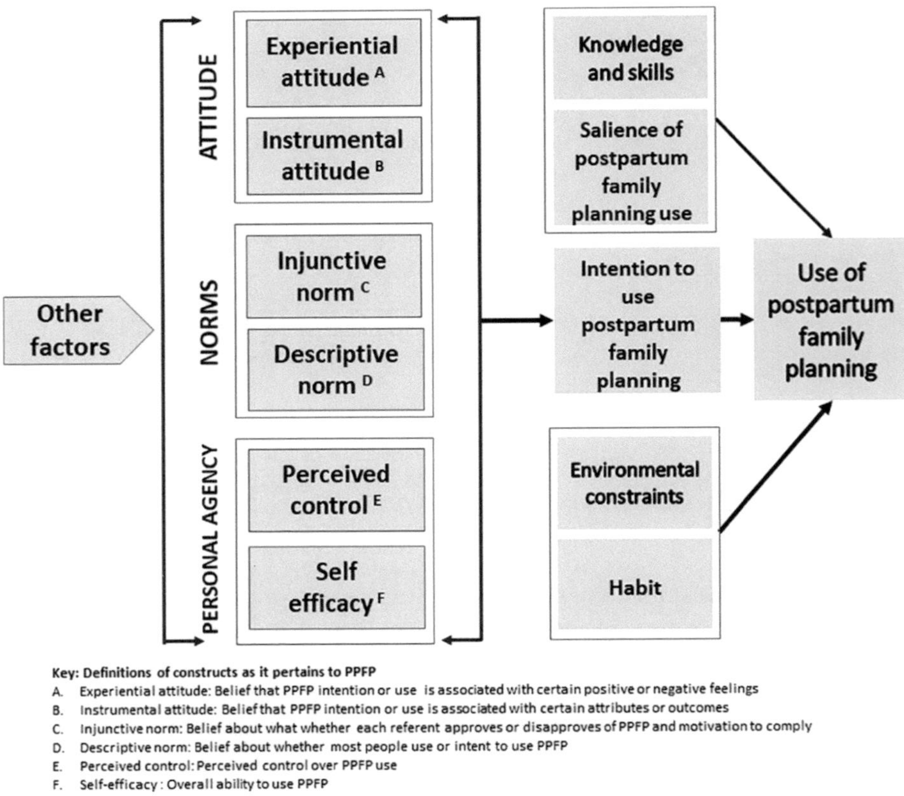

Figure 2.
Integrated behavioral model of postpartum family planning use. https://doi.org/10.1371/journal.pone.0254085.g001 [11].

injunctive norms have a negative impact and descriptive norms have a positive impact in reproductive choices. Peer norms and social norms similarly affect a person's choices in such matters. In the patriarchal society, prevalent in many LMIC reproductive decisions are not solely made by the woman. It is usually a shared family decision in which often the will and voice of the woman is the feeblest [28].

10. Administrative and community interventions to increase PPIUCD acceptance

To translate PPFP attitudes into specific messages that can be tested and refined before being scaled up into the target population, it would be useful for programs to deliberate on which myths and misconceptions are most associated with PPFP intentions in a given society and to develop culture appropriate IEC materials to persuade the target population to modify or reverse their current behavior in that respect. This can be done by popular role models and brand ambassadors with similar cultural experiences and values who would be instrumental in dispelling negative perceptions. Involvement of spouse and dominant family members in the decision-making dialog with health service providers and counselors will also contribute to reaching out to the eligible women to try PPIUCD as their long-term contraceptive option. Group counseling and peer discussions also increase confidence among users and would be users [29]. Joint decision-making by couples has also been shown to increase rates of acceptance of PPIUCD [29].

Community engagement and community-level reflection of prevailing societal practices and perceptions in order to root in PPFP into their regular reproductive lifestyle, and value system is also bound to give dividends. Facilitating young women's education and employment opportunities also empowers them to make such personalized choices, which first and foremost directly affect their health and well-being [29].

11. Barriers to PPIUCD usage at service provider level

Service providers who insert PPIUCD in the labor room, postnatal ward, or at cesarean section have varied experiences with the insertion procedure. Hence, perception regarding the efficacy and safety of PPIUCD as an option in the contraceptive basket is varied among different levels of service providers. Those who were not trained by participation in a formal training program using simulators followed by in-house training in real patients often inserted the device manually following placental delivery. Also, they were not conversant with the universal infection prevention practices and the aseptic and antiseptic precautions mandated before and during insertion of the IUCD. This may account for complications associated with PPIUCD use, which often necessitated its removal. This defeats the very purpose and benefits of PPIUCD as a long-acting reversible contraceptive (LARC). Inadequate training also leads to improper non-fundal placement of the IUCD, which is responsible for the high percentage of complete or partial expulsion intrauterine translocation causing uterine cramps or a length of IUCD thread reaching low into the vagina causing anxiety and discomfort to the woman and her spouse. Such service providers include staff nurses and auxiliary nurse midwives (ANMs) who admit lack of confidence in the procedure and therefore avoid the insertion within the stipulated time limits for postpartum insertion and postpone it for a later period. Such women who are eligible for contraception may or may not return for contraceptive provision later. This contributes to a substantial percentage of the unmet need for contraception in willing women who are vulnerable to unwanted too early subsequent pregnancies. This is a missed opportunity for providing them a reliable contraception, and they have not come back into the health care system for family planning counseling and services. Several studies have defined the health care-seeking behavior of in lower income populations as "crisis-oriented," that is they return to health facilities only if they need curative services and not for preventive services such as using a contraceptive method [30].

Similarly, at cesarean section, there is lack of uniform technique in putting in an IUCD. Some surgeons do it manually, and others use the applicator provided in the pack. What is important to be noted, especially if the device has been placed by junior surgeons who usually man the labor suites, whether the placement is at the uterine fundus in the coronal section of the cavity. Also, the direction in which the tip of the thread is pointing is also important if the tip curls up toward the fundus instead toward the external os the incidence of "missing thread" at subsequent follow-up visit becomes correspondingly high. This is a cause of worry both to the user and the service provider since in the event of irregular or heavy vaginal bleeding or infection–associated complications or if for any reason the woman insists on removal of the device the procedure becomes cumbersome. Often, a simple probing of the cervical canal with an artery forceps in the outpatient clinic is not successful in accessing the thread and frequently necessitates taking the woman to the operation theater to retrieve the device under general anesthesia often with special device retrievers. Such an intervention in a scarred uterus is itself fraught with dangers combined with the risks of G.A. This mars the confidence of the service providers who tend to eschew further intra-cesarean PPIUCD in subsequent patients. However, as for vaginal insertions, what is important is proper evidence-based training in the insertion technique rather than decrying the indication and timing of the insertion itself [31].

Apart from the faulty technique of insertion, another very important factor negatively affecting the acceptance of PPIUCD by women is the inappropriate counseling provided to them about the method in terms of timing, content, and manner of counseling. The various aspects related to PPIUCD should be discussed at antenatal visits. This is the time when women and their families are most likely to understand its various aspects and implications, voice their doubts, and concerns and make a truly informed choice. However, due to the enormous workload on the obstetricians, midwifery, and nursing staff, as well as a dearth of dedicated FP counselors who have the requisite skills and sole specific responsibility to familiarize women about their various contraceptive options many antenatal clients do not have the benefits of such structured contraceptive counseling. This causes a sharp reduction in the number of puerperal women accepting PPIUCD in the immediate postpartum period when they are still in the delivery facility. In hospitals where regular antenatal checkups are combined with repeated FP counseling the uptake of PPIUCD has been shown to be substantially higher with better long-term continuation rates also [32–35].

12. Interventions to remove service provision barriers to PPIUCD services

In order to simplify the procedure of the vaginal insertion, **dedicated PPIUCD inserters** have been devised which simplifies and ensures the fundal placement with minimal risk of uterine perforation [36, 37]. The complicated cumbersome steps of uterine axis straightening by abdominal man oeuvres followed by rotation of the IUCD into the coronal plane at the fundus are circumvented in this straightforward method. This enhances the confidence of the service providers who use it in the labor room (**Figure 3**). The total cost of the inserter including the device is less than 1US dollar, making it a very cost-effective device comparing very favorably with other methods [38]. However, it is available at some centers only, and hence insertion continues to be predominantly with the help of Kelly's placental.

Considering the long-term economic benefits of an efficient national population policy with its resultant population stabilization effects on the overall nation's economy, IUCDs are being provided free of cost at government health facilities of many LMICs such as India. Also, at several private delivery facilities, they are available at subsidized rates through social marketing schemes and strategies, thus making it affordable and accessible to a greater reach of population in such countries.

At cesarean section also it is important to emphasize to the junior surgeons and trainees who do the bulk of abdominal deliveries at the tertiary level care centers the need to ensure that the device has to be advanced through the uterine incision up to the fundus, ensuring that the device is left flat in the cavity in the coronal plane of the uterus and that its tail tip is directed toward the os. Also, once the IUCD is *in situ* at the fundus, there should be no further exploration or mopping of the uterine cavity, which would be likely to dislodge it from its proper high position. This will ensure proper placement and retention of the device as also ease of removal if it is required in any circumstances. Some surgeons have introduced techniques for intra-cesarean PPIUCD insertion to eliminate chances of expulsion of the device at any later date. One such technique is to anchor the device to the fundus with a catgut knot with the help of a straight needle passing through the fundus [37, 39].

One of the major reasons why service providers—general duty doctors and staff nurses working in labor wards, specialist obstetricians, midwives, and auxiliary nurse midwives— desist from inserting PPIUCD is lack of training and subsequent hand-holding in the early days of their post-training period. To address this issue nongovernmental agencies, such as JHpiego, United States Agency for International Development(USAID), and maternal and child health integrated program(MCHIP), have extended their support to several LMICs and pitched in with them to train obstetric personnel in correct standardized PPIUCD counseling method, insertion technique, infection prevention practices (IPP), follow-up protocol, and management

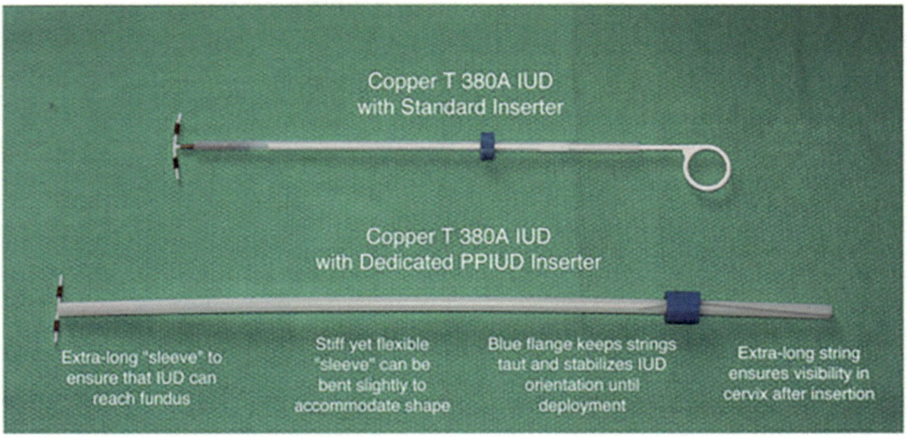

Figure 3.
Comparison between copper T 380A IUCD with standard inserter and with a dedicated PPIUCD inserter.

of post-insertion problems and complications. They have developed learning resource packages (LRP), job aids, behavior change communication (BCC), materials and toolkits in order to streamline counseling messages and insertion techniques across centers providing PPIUCD services. Training are imparted at regional and nodal centers initially to some medical and nursing staff of a delivery site. Their competency is determined on the basis of checklists of the various competencies; they have achieved in order to effectively and safely provide PPIUCD services at their workplace. Post-training these trained personnel start PPIUCD services at their workplace. A cascade effect of such formal training ensues as the few personnel who attend such formal training at nodal and regional training centers go back to their parent institutions and are in a position to do in-house training and supervision in PPIUCD counseling and insertion of their work colleagues there. Such initiatives have been shown to increase rates of PPIUCD acceptance and continuation rates with very low rates of reported expulsion (2.5%), infection (0.9%), and removals (4.2%). The efforts of such agencies, which extend technical training support, are laudable since they continue to support them at their workplace. They maintain their communication lines with them so that in the event of any difficulty they feel supported. This is a very important confidence-building measure for the staff especially those working in remote isolated places [33].

Maintenance of quality performance standards is done by regular audits of the PPIUCD documentation and records. During training service providers are also trained in record-keeping related to PPIUCD service. This helps in assessment of service delivery quality in terms of client follow-up data relating to expulsions, infection, request for removals, and overall patient satisfaction with respect to the device, service provision center, and the service provider. Client follow-up is done either at the time of their follow-up visits at the health care facility or telephonically if they do not report back. Monitoring of PPIUCD programs through audits helps gap analysis of the services being currently provided at a center, and how services could be improved both in terms of quality and number of insertions.

Demand generation can be enhanced by hiring and training dedicated counselors who are provided with job aids and IEC materials, which have been customized to culturally and linguistically appropriate standards. A cafeteria approach during family planning counseling sessions will allow women to make a truly informed contraceptive choice. PPIUCD has the potential to satisfy the requirements of many primipara and multipara women following delivery.

Supply management in government facilities needs to be bolstered to prevent stock-outs. This will ensure that supply meets demand, otherwise, it may lead to unmet need for contraception for women who are keen to prevent pregnancies. In women seeking contraceptive provision in private facilities vouchers, social marketing campaigns, and mobile service delivery systems can ensure availability and affordability for them.

An increase in number of service providers trained in PPIUCD counseling and insertion skills can be done by regular training-of-trainers sessions. Updated guidelines and incorporation of PPIUCD in regular medical curricula will also improve the service delivery system by increasing the number of service providers.

13. Conclusion

Despite WHO evidence-based recommendations of birth–spacing of at least three years, PPFP remains a neglected area in obstetrics, especially in developing countries with burgeoning population. However, during the last two decades, there has a resurgence of interest globally in the use of the IUCD during the immediate postpartum period within forty-eight hours of delivery when the woman is still within the delivery site. FIGO's initiative in popularizing it in six LMICs as a viable PPFP option in the contraceptive basket has been strengthened by nongovernmental organizations, such as JHpiego, USAID, PSI, and MCHIP. They are collectively extending technical and training support to various governments in southeast Asia and sub-Saharan Africa who have recognized the immense potential in promoting their respective national population control policies and programs.

As for any program launched on a widespread scale, PPIUCD FP program also requires robust field data pertaining to the users, as well as service providers, administrative, and budgetary cells in order to evaluate, whether it is performing satisfactorily as regards its expected primary and secondary related outcomes. Accumulated data from systematic reviews on the topic indicate that the main barriers and challenges in increasing acceptance and continuation of PPIUCD are low awareness, and hence demand for its use by prospective clients. This is coupled with low motivation, poor counseling and technical skills, and confidence of service providers in its insertion. Other issues of concern relate to supply chain, which has to be addressed by policy makers and health and FP budget planners.

From whatever data that have accumulated from diverse LMIC populations PPIUCD despite its "below expected" success in lowering TFR remains a promising PPFP option for eligible women provided it is backed up by proper IEC strategies coupled with training in quality counseling and insertion skills and practice by the service providers. Individual prejudices based on limited personal experience and opinion need to be aggressively curtailed in order to prevent reduction in rates of user acceptance of a very useful contraceptive method. Future research in the individual country specific contexts should be directed at obviating such obstacles for the wider use of this effective PPFP method, which has the benefit of being an extremely effective LARC, which compares favorably with permanent birth limiting methods.

Author details

Tripti Sinha
Department of Obstetrics and Gynecology, Sri Krishna Medical College, Muzaffarpur, Bihar, India

*Address all correspondence to: triptisinha0304@gmail.com

IntechOpen

© 2023 The Author(s). Licensee IntechOpen. This chapter is distributed under the terms of the Creative Commons Attribution License (http://creativecommons.org/licenses/by/3.0), which permits unrestricted use, distribution, and reproduction in any medium, provided the original work is properly cited.

References

[1] Dev R, Kohler P, Feder M, Unger JA, Woods NF, Drake AL. A systematic review and meta-analysis of postpartum contraceptive use among women in low- and middle-income countries. Reproductive Health: BioMedical Central Ltd. 2019;**16**(154):1-17. DOI: 10.1186/s12978-019-0824-4

[2] Gadisa TB, Michael MW, Reda MM, Aboma BD. Early resumption of postpartumsexual intercourse and its associated risk factorsamong married postpartum women who visitedpublic hospitals of Jimma zone, SouthwestEthiopia: A cross-sectional study. PLoS One. 2021;**16**(3):e0247769. DOI: 10.1371/journal.pone.0247769

[3] World Health Organisation. Programming Strategies for Postpartum Family Planning. Geneva, Switzerland: World Health Organization; 2013 Available from: https://apps.who.int/iris/handle/10665/9368

[4] World Health Organization & United States. Agency for International Development. Programming Strategies for Postpartum Family Planning. Geneva: WHO; 2013. Available from: https://apps.who.int/iris/handle/10665/93680

[5] ACCESS-FP Program. FP needs during the extended PP period, analysis of Pakistan DHS 2006-07. Jhpiego: National Institute of Population Studies (NIPS) [Pakistan], and Macro International Inc. 2008. Pakistan Demographic and Health Survey 2006-07. Islamabad, Pakistan: National Institute of Population Studies and Macro International Inc; 2009. Available from: https://www.k4health.org/sites/default/files/Pakistan%202006-2007%20DHS%20Reanalysis%20for%20PPFP_Final_0.pdf [Accessed July 7, 2017

[6] WHO Global Code of Practice on International Recruitment of Health Personnel Implementation Strategy Report 2011–Pakistan. Pakistan Nursing Council. Islamabad. Economic Survey of Pakistan 2013-2014.

[7] Black RE, Levin C, Walker N, Chou D, Liu L, Temmerman M. Reproductive, maternal, newborn, and child health: Key messages from disease control priorities. The Lancet. 2016;**2016**:2811-2824. DOI: 10.1016/S0140-6736(16)00738-)

[8] Healthy People 2020. Available from: https://www.healthypeople.gov/2020/topics-objectives/topic/family-planning

[9] Huang YM, Merkatz R, Kang JZ. Postpartum unintended pregnancy and contraception practice among rural-tourban migrant women in Shanghai. Contraception. 2012;**86**:731-738. DOI: 10.1016/j.contraception.2012.05.007

[10] Report of a Technical Consultation on Birth Spacing. 2005. https://www.who.int/maternal_child_adolescent/documents/birth_spacing05/en/ [Accessed: September 2, 2019].

[11] Cleland J, Lenka MA, Daniele BM. The promotion of intrauterine contraception in low- and middle-income countries: A narrative review. Contraception. 2017;**95**:519-528

[12] Makins A, Taghinejadi N, Sethi M, Machiyama K, Munganyizi P, Odongo E, et al. FIGO postpartum intrauterine device initiative: Complicationrates across six countries. International Journal of Gynecology and Obstetrics. 2018;**143**(Suppl. 1):20-27

[13] Fatima P, Arefa Hossain AA, Dewan F, Nash S, Sethi M. Impact of

contraceptive counselling training among counselors participating in the FIGO postpartum intrauterine device initiative in Bangladesh. International Journal of Gynecology and Obstetrics. 2018;**143**(Suppl. 1):49-55

[14] Muganyizi PS, Kimario G, Ponsian P, Howard K, Sethi M, Makins A. Clinical outcomes of postpartum intrauterine devices inserted by midwives in Tanzania. International Journal of Gynecology and Obstetrics. 2018;**143**(Suppl. 1):38-42

[15] Deepal SW, Senanayeke L, Pushpananda U, Perera RGY, Lanerolle S, Sanjeeva S, et al. Four years of the FIGO postpartum intrauterine device initiative in Sri Lanka: Pilot initiative to national policy. International Journal of Gynecology and Obstetrics. 2018;**143**(Suppl. 1):28-32

[16] Thapa K, Dhital R, Karki YB, Rajbhandari S, Amatya S, Pande S, et al. Institutionalizing postpartum family planning and postpartum intrauterine device services in Nepal: Role of training and mentorship. International Journal of Gynecology and Obstetrics. 2018;**143**(Suppl. 1):43-48

[17] USAID J. Postpartum Intrauterine Contraceptive Device (PPIUD) Services. Baltimore, Maryland: Learner's Handbook; 2010. Available from: https://toolkits.knowledgesuccess.org/sites/default/files/ppiud_learners_guide_update.pdf

[18] WHO. Medical Eligibility Criteria for Contraceptive Use. 5th ed. Geneva, Switzerland: WHO Press; 2015. https://apps.who.int/iris/bitstream/handle/10665/181468/9789241549158_eng.pdf?sequence=9

[19] Executive summary. WHO. 2015. https://apps.who.int/iris/bitstream/handle/10665/181468/9789241549158_eng.pdf?sequence=9

[20] Rosa Bolling K, Schoendorf J, Pisa F, Gomez-Espinosa E, Kistler K, Maiese B, et al. Utilisation, effectiveness, and safety of immediate postpartum intrauterine device insertion: A systematic literature review. BMJ Sexual Reproductive Health. 2022;**0**:1-30. DOI: 10.1136/bmjsrh-2022-201579

[21] Kanakuze CA, Kaye DK, Musabirema P, et al. Factors associated with the uptake of immediate postpartum intrauterine contraceptive devices (PPIUCD) in Rwanda: A mixed methods study. BMC PregnancyChildbirth. 2020;**20**:650. DOI: 10.1186/s12884-020-03337-5

[22] Mark KP, Leistner CE, Garcia JR. Impact of contraceptive type on sexual desire of women and of men partnered to contraceptive users. Journal of Sexual Medicine. 2016;**13**(9):1359-1368. DOI: 10.1016/j.jsxm.2016.06.011

[23] NHS. Intrauterine device (IUD). Available from: https://www.nhs.uk/conditions/contraception/iud-coil/

[24] Maternal and Child Health Integrated Program (MCHIP); Population Services International (PSI). PPIUD Services: Start-up to Scale-up Regional Meeting Burkina Faso: February 3-5, 2014 meeting report. Washington (DC): MCHIP; 2014. Co-published by PSI, 2014. Available from: http://www.mchip.net/node/2793

[25] United Nations (UN), Department of Economic and Social Affairs, Population Division. World Contraceptive Use 2015. New York: UN; 2015. Available from: http://www.un.org/en/development/desa/population/publications/dataset/contraception/wcu2015.shtml

[26] Singh S. Facilitators and barriers in acceptance of postpartum intrauterine contraceptive devices in Bihar. Indian Journal of Obstetrics and Gynecology Research. 2022;**9**(4):506-514

[27] Gage AJ, Wood FE, Akilimali PZ. Perceived norms, personal agency, and postpartum family planning intentions among first time mothers age 15-24 years in Kinshasa: A cross-sectional analysis. PLoS One. 2021;**16**(7):e0254085. DOI: 10.1371/journal.pone.0254085

[28] Hutchinson PL, Anaba U, Abegunde D, Okoh M, Hewett PC, Johansson EW. Understanding family planning outcomes in northwestern Nigeria: Analysis and modeling of social and behavior change factors. BMC Public Health. 2021;**21**:116

[29] Sebastian MP, Khan ME, Kumari K, Idnani R. Increasing postpartum contraception in rural India : Evaluation of a community based behavior change communication intervention. International Perspectives on Sexual and Reproductive Health. 2012;**38**(2):68-77

[30] Husain S, Husain S, Izhar R. Women's decision versus couples' decision on using postpartum intra-uterine contraceptives. Eastern Mediterranean Health Journal. 2019;**25**(5):322-330. DOI: 10.26719/emhj.18.043

[31] Price NL, Hawkins K. A conceptual framework for the social analysis of reproductive health. Journal of Health, Population, and Nutrition. 2007;**25**(1):24-36

[32] Gupta N, Sinha R, Mangal A. Knowledge, attitude and practice study on immediate postpartum intrauterine contraceptive device method of family planning. International Journal of Community Medicine and Public Health. 2017;**4**(8):2981

[33] Zafar Z, Habib H, Kols A, Enriquito FA, Lu R, Schuster A. Reinvigorating postpartum intrauterine contraceptive device use in Pakistan: An observational assessment of competency based training of health providers using low-cost simulation models. BMC Medical Education. 2019;**19**:261. DOI: 10.1186/s12909-019-1683-y

[34] Pradhan E, Canning D, Shah IH, Puri M, Pearson E, Thapa K, et al. Integrating postpartum contraceptive counseling and IUD insertion services into maternity care in Nepal: Results from stepped-wedge randomized controlled trial. Reproductive Health. 2019;**16**(1):69. DOI: 10.1186/s12978-019-0738-1

[35] Raghuwanshi M, Agrawal S, Singh BK, Khatik N. Postpartum intrauterine contraceptive device: Effect of antenatal versus postpartum counselling in acceptance of postpartum intrauterine contraceptive device. International Journal of Reproduction, Contraception, Obstetrics and Gynecology. 2020;**9**:3742-3748

[36] Pradeep MR, Nayana DH. Study of knowledge, attitude and acceptance of PPIUCD in antenatal mothers. The New Indian Journal of Obstetrics and Gynecology. 2019;**6**(1):42-44

[37] Singh S, Das V, Agarwal A, Dewan R, Mittal P, Bhamrah R, et al. A dedicated postpartum intrauterine device inserter: Pilot experience and proof of concept. Global Health Science Practice. 2016;**4**(1):132-140. DOI: 10.9745/GHSP-D-15-00355

[38] Shukla S, Tyagi M, Gupta S, Yadav L. Compare ease of insertion,

visibility of strings and continuation rate of post-partum intrauterine copper device insertion by long inserter versus with the help of Kelly's forceps. International Journal of Reproductive and Contraceptive Obstetrics and Gynecology. 2021;**10**:74-77

[39] Tjahjanto H, Haryuni IT. Hang-up IUD, new technique for suturing CuT-380A IUD to uterine fundus in immediate post-placental insertion during cesarean delivery: Twelve months follow up. Indonesian Journal of Obstetrics and Gynecology. 2014;**2**(31):132-139

Section 2

Postnatal Issues

Chapter 3

Perspective Chapter: Contemporary Challenges in Postnatal Care in Low- and Middle-Income Countries

Amen A. Bawazir

Abstract

The postnatal phase is the first six weeks after delivery and is a critical time for mothers, newborns, and other caregivers as a highly neglected phase of a transition period. Almost all maternal and neonatal deaths occur in low- and middle-income countries, where fewer services are provided for mothers after the delivery period, which constitutes a tremendous challenge facing mothers in these countries. Barriers were markedly observed in low-and middle-income countries as a result of financial constraints, distance from the health center, poor programming for postnatal care, negative childbirth experiences, and cultural constraints. Moreover, the unproper advocacy of contraceptive use during the postpartum period impacts prolonged interpregnancy intervals and indirectly increases postpartum complications mainly in low- and middle-income countries. The importance of the quality of postnatal care was frequently addressed to answer the required interventions that should be implemented at the level of healthcare facilities, household, and community levels as part of the process of reducing the impact of postnatal complications, disabilities, and maternal mortality.

Keywords: women, postpartum, mothers, maternal mortality, reproductive program

1. Introduction

The World Health Organization (WHO) has defined the postnatal phase as the first six weeks after delivery, which is a critical time for mothers, newborns, partners, parents, caregivers, and families; however, this period of significant transition remains the most neglected phase in quality maternal and newborn health care [1].

Therefore, this chapter will discuss the impact of postnatal care in low- and middle-income countries and the main challenges they face. Moreover, the chapter will highlight the importance of the quality of postnatal care required at the level of the facility, household, and community levels as part of the process of reducing the impact of postnatal complications. Such services should be provided for every woman on this globe with more empathy for those in low- and middle-income countries. In addition, this chapter will address the quality of care needed based on the positive

IntechOpen

postnatal experience, factors influencing the positive birth, and finally the role of contraceptives in reducing maternal complications.

As per the use of the World Bank Atlas for the year 2023 to define low- and middle-income countries are those with a Gross National Income (GNI) per capita between $1086 and $4255 [2].

Despite the global achievements found during the implementation of the Millennium Development Goals and impressive reductions in maternal and under-5 mortality rates, neonatal mortality reduction continues to lag behind [2]. Moreover, maternal and neonatal mortality and morbidity burdens remain unacceptably high, and opportunities to increase maternal well-being and support nurturing newborn care have not been fully utilized [1]. Therefore, the global health community has worked hard to make good achievements over the past decades and has continuous challenges in the future to accomplish the sustainable development goals (SDGs) by the end of 2030 [3].

2. Definitions

Postnatal care (PNC) ensures early assessments for pregnancy danger signs during the postpartum period and is to be provided within 24 hours of birth, 48–72 hours, 7–14 days, and 6 weeks after birth [1]. Therefore, postnatal care services are a fundamental component of the maternal, newborn, and childcare continuum and are key to achieving the sustainable development goals (SDGs) on reproductive, maternal, and child health, including targets to reduce maternal mortality rates and end preventable deaths of newborns [1]. Moreover, in line with the SDGs, postnatal care efforts must expand beyond the optimum coverage by maternal services and survival alone to include quality of care.

Although postnatal care services are a fundamental element of the continuum of essential obstetric care and were implemented to play a role in decreasing maternal and neonatal morbidity and mortality, particularly in low- and middle-income countries still, almost 40% of women experience complications after delivery and an estimated 15% develop potentially life-threatening problems [4–6]. As almost all (99%) of maternal and neonatal deaths occur in developing countries [7], inequality is a prominent matter among high-income and low- and middle-income countries where almost three out of four women had ≥one symptom (73.5%), abnormalities on clinical examination (71.3%), or laboratory investigation (73.5%) after delivery mainly in the postnatal period [8]. Moreover, maternal morbidity was not limited to a core “at-risk” group; only 1.2% of women had a combination of four morbidities.

3. How to reach a positive postnatal experience?

A positive postnatal experience is recognized as a significant endpoint for all women giving birth and their newborns, laying the platform for improved short- and long-term health and well-being [9]. It is also defined as when women, newborns, partners, parents, caregivers, and families receive information, reassurance, and support consistently from motivated health workers; where a resourced and flexible health system recognizes the needs of women and babies and respects their cultural context. Moreover, the positive birth experience promotes a sense of achievement, enhances a feeling of self-worth, and facilitates confidence; all of which are important for a healthy adaptation to motherhood and psychological growth [10]. Understanding what constitutes a positive birth experience is critical to providing maternity care that meets childbearing women's individual needs, preferences, and priorities. Likely wise, any satisfaction with birth has been associated with several factors and the Psychosocial dimensions of care have been shown to influence women's overall assessment. Individualized emotional support empowers women and increases the possibility of a positive birth experience [11].

Therefore, the human reproductive program initiated by the World Health Organization has developed a comprehensive set of recommendations for care during the antenatal and postnatal period, focusing on the essential package that all women and newborns should receive, with due attention to the quality of care, that is, the provision and experience of care and management of postnatal complications [1].

4. Factors influencing positive birth and postnatal care

It was found that most women lacked awareness about the services given in a postnatal clinic and long waiting times, and cultural beliefs were among the factors that affected utilization of postnatal care in many countries with severe situations in low-income countries. The care during puerperium for the woman hasan influence on maternal health if the woman does not attend postnatal care services and yet this is one of the most important maternal health-care services for not only prevention of impairment and disabilities but also reduction of maternal mortality.

One of the most important events in a woman's life is to giving birth, which is a highly individual experience [12]. Childbirth by itself is an experience of how first-time mothers will develop good self-esteem [13], positive feelings for the baby, an easier adjustment to the motherhood role [14, 15], future childbirth experiences [11], and better acceptance of the maternal role [16].

Being with positive birth is also influenced by other factors including the sociodemographic factors from one country to another. For example, in high-income countries, women's birth experiences changed over time, and most became more positive after 1 year [10]. Factors associated with a very positive birth experience and reduction of the impact of postnatal complications were related to women's prenatal attitudes, intrapartum procedures, pain relief used, and care received during labor and birth. Many of these factors were struggled to find low-income countries where there are poor services, lack of preparatory sessions for mother and her partner, lack of access to healthcare services on time, and cost-wise factor. Therefore, negative and traumatic birth experiences are a marked trend in women living in low-income countries mainly during prenatal and intrapartum practices [17].

The rate of psychological birth trauma including poor maternal feelings was also found high, as poor quality of maternity care and, consequently, chronic psychological complications, receiving of inaccurate information, and inadequate feeling of respect, all were also found high in low- and middle-income countries compared to high-income countries [18]. Some description of such conditions as due to lack of adequate and timely procedures beginning with admission to postpartum care resulted in poor quality of care for the mother and her baby, ranging from negligence to severe complications [19]. Sociocultural barriers are also considered to play role in hindering mothers from receiving care in hospitals [20]. For instance, women preferred not to be examined by male health providers, for cultural reasons preferred a particular position in which to deliver, or for religious reasons did not divulge information that was needed for their care [21, 22]. Moreover, some communities in low-and middle-income countries reported mistreatment of mothers during labor, violation of women's rights, and a notable barrier to institutional delivery [18].

5. Trends in contraceptive use

According to the WHO, postpartum family planning (PPFP) is defined as the prevention of unintended pregnancy and closely spaced pregnancies through the first 12 months following childbirth [23]. The proper practice of contraceptives during the postpartum period has its impact on prolonging interpregnancy interval and indirectly reduces postpartum complications and other consequences [24]. Therefore, contraceptives help in the prevention of unwanted pregnancies among couples and, therefore, promote planned family size and time of birth for improved reproductive well-being of the women. Voluntary family planning practices include the promotion of maternal and child health, human rights, population and development, and environmental sustainability and development of a nation. However, the use of contraceptives was found with marked variation between developed and developing nations, across nations, and within nations. Despite the United Nations (2015) report on the trend of contraceptive use among women of the reproductive age group, who are either married or in a union, in almost all regions of the world reached up to 64% [23]. At the end of the millennium development goals, the United Nations report showed that contraceptive use was much lower in the least developed countries with an estimate of 40.0% with the African continent had the lowest estimated at 33.0% [24]. In Nigeria for example, only 14.5% of women use modern contraceptive methods according to the estimation from the national population commission [25]. Moreover, over 83% of women were not using any form of contraceptives in 2018 with a geographical variation within the country [26]. Regional averages hide some of the more dramatic variations in contraceptive sources at the country level [27]. More than half of women in low- and middle-income countries using modern contraception go to private sector sources than public sources [28].

The sustainable development goals (SDGs) target 3.7 calls on all countries "by 2030 to ensure universal access to sexual and reproductive health-care services, including for family planning, information and education, and the integration of reproductive health into national strategies and programs" [29]. The assessment of progress toward this target requires monitoring of key family planning indicators, including the range and types of contraceptive methods used [27]. There are several barriers to using effective methods in low- and middle-income countries including the desire for more children, partner disapproval of contraceptive use, religious and cultural bias, educational qualification of women, lack of knowledge on contraceptives, and wealth index [30]. Additional factors reported, such as concerns about the side effects of contraceptive methods, women's or their family's opposition to contraception, lack of access to supplies and services, and especially financial barriers, are often reported [31]. Consequently, a trend of high family sizes of up to seven or above is common in many regions of low- and middle-income countries.

6. Unmet need for family planning due to poor postpartum period education

The unmet need for family planning as a crucial factor in determining equity among women at the postnatal time is almost liked mutual with the use of contraceptives. Mothers, since the first days after delivery, should be equipped with proper information on the use of contraceptives to avoid the condition unmet for family planning and arrange their next pregnancy with adequate time [29]. At least one in ten married or in-union women in most regions of the world have an unmet need for family planning. Worldwide, in 2015, 12% of married or in-union women are estimated to have had an unmet need for family planning; that is, they wanted to stop or delay childbearing but were not using any method of contraception. Estimates of the percentage of women aged 15–49 years who use contraception or who have an unmet need for family planning, by region, for the year 2020 showed that only 35.9% of women in Northern Africa and West Asia compared to 60% in Europe and Northern America [29]. The level was much higher, 22%, in the least developed countries. Many of these countries are in sub-Saharan Africa, which is also the region where the unmet need was highest (24%), double the world average in 2015 [24]. Unmet need is generally higher among younger women in the poorest households and among those who have less education and live in rural areas. Despite efforts and availability of contraceptives in low- and middle-income countries, uptake continues to be low because of several barriers [32, 33].

7. Role of adverse events (AEs)

Good postnatal care is crucial to prevent adverse maternal and neonatal outcomes and provide support during motherhood adjustment for first-time mothers. Adverse events (AEs) are outcomes of treatments below the current expected medical standard that result in temporary or permanent harm to patients. Unplanned, adverse events during labor or delivery may generate a negative response during the early postpartum period, resulting in disruption of usual functioning and mood. Most maternal and neonatal adverse events occur in the immediate postnatal period [34]. The provision of evidence-based postnatal care with adequate quality during this period is vital to ensure uncomplicated recovery of the mother and the baby. In some low- and middle-income countries, AEs episodes were identified among both mothers and newborns with an overall prevalence of 12.7% [35].

High levels of maternal depressive symptoms during the postnatal period are associated with parenting, infant attachment, behavioral problems, and cognition [36]. In many low- and middle-income countries, woman's dissatisfaction status with their own childbirth experience was less likely reported, however, the severe depressive state could be noticed as accompanying emotional unwillingness to have another baby due to such malpractices occurring either in healthcare settings or in-home births [32, 33]. Such preventable adverse events were reported as complicating the postnatal period including the postpartum length of stay for more than 3 days after vaginal birth and delayed intervention in case of postnatal hemorrhage (PPH) with a decision-delivery time of more than 30 minutes [37]. Prolonged (labor) second stage was found strongly associated as a risk factor during childbirth with multiparous mothers, the use of uterine fundus pressure as one of the intervention methods during labor was associated with AEs among mothers [35, 38].

Many women recognized the specific challenges of the postnatal period and emphasized the need for emotional and psychosocial support in addition to clinical care. Postnatal care programs and related research should consider these multiple drivers and multifaceted needs, and the holistic postpartum needs of women and their families should be studied in a wider range of settings [32].

8. Barriers

Improvements in the services related to postpartum were noticed worldwide despite the variation between countries or within the country regions. However, barriers were markedly observed in low- and middle-income countries where postnatal care utilization was low at village levels and where 70% of the mothers were settled down [39]. Financial constraints, distance from the health center, poor programming for postnatal care, women's experience during childbirth, cultural constraints, mother and family members' health literacy on postnatal care, feeling that postnatal visits were not necessary, sociocultural beliefs, and practices, whichhindered mothers from utilizing postnatal care and from having adequate nutritional intake during the postnatal period [39, 40]. Other factors were related to the health system such as insufficient staff, poor reception of clients, lack of trust and confidentiality between clients and health care providers, lack of sensitization and information, and midwives' workloads [41]. In addition, patient-centered care practices, capacities to conduct postnatal information, education, and counseling are considered among the main barriers to the use of proper postnatal care mainly in remote areas of low- and middle-income nations [39, 42].

9. Advocate for best practices in the postpartum period

Changing behavior to promote a positive attitude in low- and middle-income countries is an element that should be practiced at the base of primary healthcare settings and referred obstetric hospitals. The duty of the healthcare services is to provide adequate care for women during the postpartum period. Designing effective interventions based on practically sound activities related to the postpartum period, accepted by the local communities and adopted to sustain the well-being of women and their families is a crucial step to maximize engagement and outcomes in these communities.

Such required activities and practices focus on behavioral change and address factors related to effective knowledge, attitudes, and norms as part of the interventions. The World Health Organization guidelines addressing postpartum care are well-defined and able to apply and accommodate such communities with low resources [41]. These interventions often complement and enhance the role played by services such as health promotion and education for health care services like family planning, antenatal care, delivery in a skilled birth attendant, and postnatal care [25, 42]. Social and behavior change interventions are critical to ensure that populations that are most in need can access available services and products. This is often achievable through a well-planned and systematically implemented social and behavior change intervention that is based on formative research. In addition, a good, strategic plan that is based on identifying the barriers, mode of communication to the population, and tailored messages to address specific behaviors to enhance the proper practices of women, family, and healthcare services toward improving the impact of postnatal practices in low- and middle-income countries is crucial [41]. However, implementing best-practice for postnatal activities may require a better understanding of the situation by the health authorities and relevant stockholders working in the area of health services and care. In addition, it is wise to design a focused strategy, developing interventions and materials, and implementing, monitoring, evaluating, and adjusting the planned strategies [43]. Various activities could be included in this planning strategy such as raising awareness, reducing misinformation, and addressing barriers to various lifesaving and health-promoting interventions among individuals, families, and communities.

10. Conclusion

This chapter discussed the impact of postnatal care in low- and middle-income countries and the main challenges they face. Moreover, the importance of the quality of postnatal care was also addressed as well as the required interventions that should be implemented at the level of the facility, household, and community levels as part of the process of reducing the impact of postnatal complications. Such services should be provided for every woman on this globe with more empathy for those in low- and middle-income countries.

As almost all maternal and neonatal deaths occur in developing countries, inequality is a prominent matter among high-income and low- and middle-income countries where fewer services were reported after delivery in the postnatal period. The care during puerperium for the woman has an influence on maternal health, which is considered the most important maternal health-care service not only for prevention of impairment and disabilities but also for reduction of maternal mortality.

Barriers were markedly observed in low- and middle-income countries where postnatal care utilization was low as a result of financial constraints, distance from the health center, poor programming for postnatal care, women's experience during childbirth, cultural constraints, and many others. Other factors related to the health system, such as insufficient staff, poor reception of clients, and lack of trust and confidentiality between clients and healthcare providers, were considered among the barrier to giving attention to postpartum care.

Guidelines and recommendations on a reproductive program initiated by the World Health Organization have developed a comprehensive set of plans for care during the antenatal and postnatal period, focusing on the essential package that all women and newborns should receive, with due attention to the quality of care, that is, the provision of and experience of care and management of postnatal complications. The contraceptives for the family program were linked with women's health, which helps in the prevention of unwanted pregnancies among couples and therefore promotes planned family size and time of birth for improved reproductive well-being of the women.

Strengthening health systems is crucial for improving the quality of care for mothers and neonates. To increase the responsiveness of systems and improve quality, it is essential to improve infrastructure and equipment; access to energy, water, and sanitation; and recruitment, training, and retention of health workers.

Author details

Amen A. Bawazir[1,2]

1 Faculty of Medicine and Health Sciences, University of Aden, Yemen

2 College of Medicine, AlMaaref University, Riyadh, Saudi Arabia

*Address all correspondence to: bawazir56@gmail.com

IntechOpen

© 2023 The Author(s). Licensee IntechOpen. This chapter is distributed under the terms of the Creative Commons Attribution License (http://creativecommons.org/licenses/by/3.0), which permits unrestricted use, distribution, and reproduction in any medium, provided the original work is properly cited.

References

[1] WHO. WHO recommendations on maternal and newborn care for a positive postnatal experience. Geneva: World Health Organization; 2022

[2] Lawn JE, Blencowe H, Oza S, You D, Lee AC, Waiswa P, et al. Every Newborn: Progress, priorities, and potential beyond survival. The Lancet. 2014;**384**(9938):189-205

[3] Barclay H, Dattler R, Lau K, Abdelrhim S, Marshall A, Feeney L. Sustainable Development Goals: A SRHR CSO Guide for National Implementation. London, United Kingdom: International Planned Parenthood Federation; 2015

[4] Gabrysch S, Campbell OM. Still too far to walk: Literature review of the determinants of delivery service use. BMC Pregnancy and Childbirth. 2009;**9**(1):1-18

[5] Langlois ÉV, Miszkurka M, Zunzunegui MV, Ghaffar A, Ziegler D, Karp I. Inequities in postnatal care in low-and middle-income countries: A systematic review and meta-analysis. Bulletin of the World Health Organization. 2015;**93**:259-270G

[6] Mosiur Rahman M, Haque SE, Sarwar ZM. Factors affecting the utilisation of postpartum care among young mothers in Bangladesh. Health & Social Care in the Community. 2011;**19**(2):138-147

[7] WHO. The trend in maternal mortality: 1990 to 2010: WHO, UNICEF, UNFPA, and The World Bank estimate. Geneva: World Health Organization; 2012

[8] McCauley M, Madaj B, White SA, Dickinson F, Bar-Zev S, Aminu M, et al. Burden of physical, psychological and social ill-health during and after pregnancy among women in India, Pakistan, Kenya and Malawi. BMJ Global Health. 2018;**3**(3):e000625

[9] Hosseini Tabaghdehi M, Keramat A, Kolahdozan S, Shahhosseini Z, Moosazadeh M, Motaghi Z. Positive childbirth experience: A qualitative study. Nursing Open. 2020;**7**(4):1233-1238

[10] Hildingsson I, Johansson M, Karlström A, Fenwick J. Factors associated with a positive birth experience: An exploration of swedish women's experiences. International Journal of Childbirth. 2013;**3**(3):153-164

[11] Nilsson L, Thorsell T, Hertfelt Wahn E, Ekström A. Factors influencing positive birth experiences of first-time mothers. Nursing Research and Practice. 2013;**2013**

[12] Martins ACM, Giugliani ERJ, Nunes LN, Bizon AMBL, de Senna AFK, Paiz JC, et al. Factors associated with a positive childbirth experience in Brazilian women: A cross-sectional study. Women and Birth. 2021;**34**(4):337-345

[13] Galle A, Van Parys A-S, Roelens K, Keygnaert I. Expectations and satisfaction with antenatal care among pregnant women with a focus on vulnerable groups: A descriptive study in Ghent. BMC Women's Health. 2015;**15**(1):1-12

[14] McNamara J, Risi A, Bird AL, Townsend ML, Herbert JS. The role of pregnancy acceptability in maternal mental health and bonding during pregnancy. BMC Pregnancy and Childbirth. 2022;**22**(1):1-10

[15] Demirezen RD, Aksoy OD. Effects of identification of a motherhood role

and pregnancy on marital adjustment. International Journal of Caring Sciences. 2021;**14**(3):1611

[16] Fasanghari M, Kordi M, Asgharipour N. Effect of maternal role training program based on Mercer theory on maternal self-confidence of primiparous women with unplanned pregnancy. Journal of Education and Health Promotion. 2019;**2019**:8

[17] Gage AD, Carnes F, Blossom J, Aluvaala J, Amatya A, Mahat K, et al. In low-and middle-income countries, is delivery in high-quality obstetric facilities geographically feasible? Health Affairs. 2019;**38**(9):1576-1584

[18] Wassihun B, Zeleke S. Compassionate and respectful maternity care during facility based child birth and women's intent to use maternity service in Bahir Dar, Ethiopia. BMC Pregnancy and Childbirth. 2018;**18**(1):1-9

[19] Tefera M, Assefa N, Roba KT, Gedefa L, Brewis A, Schuster RC. Women's hospital birth experiences in Harar, eastern Ethiopia: A qualitative study using Roy's Adaptation Model. BMJ Open. 2022;**12**(7):e055250

[20] Munabi-Babigumira S, Glenton C, Lewin S, Fretheim A, Nabudere H. Factors that influence the provision of intrapartum and postnatal care by skilled birth attendants in low-and middle-income countries: A qualitative evidence synthesis. Cochrane Database of Systematic Reviews. 2017;**2017**:11

[21] Khalaf I, Abu-Moghli F, Callister L, Mahadeen A, Kaawa K, Zomot A. Jordanian health care providers' perceptions of post-partum health care. International Nursing Review. 2009;**56**(4):442-449

[22] Nyondo-Mipando AL, Chirwa M, Kumitawa A, Salimu S, Nkhoma J, Chimuna TJ, et al. Uptake of, Barriers and Enablers to the Utilization of Postnatal Care Services in Thyolo. Malawi; 2022

[23] Fink G, Sudfeld CR, Danaei G, Ezzati M, Fawzi WW. Scaling-up access to family planning may improve linear growth and child development in low and middle income countries. PLoS One. 2014;**9**(7):e102391

[24] UN/DESAPD. Trends in Contraceptive Use Worldwide 2015. New York: United Nations; 2015

[25] Franco A. Scaling up contraception through social and behavior change intervention in low and middle-income countries. In: Amarin ZO, editor. Studies in Family Planning. London, UK: IntechOpen; 2022

[26] NPC. Nigeria demographic and health survey 2013. Abuja, Nigeria: National Population Commission, ICF International; 2013

[27] United Nations, Department of Economic and Social Affairs, Population Division (2019). Contraceptive Use by Method. 2019: Data Booklet. New York. (USA) (ST/ESA/SER.A/435) http://creativecommons.org/licenses/by/3.0/igo/

[28] Bradley SE, Shiras T. Where Women Access Contraception in 36 Low-and Middle-Income Countries and Why It Matters. Global Health: Science and Practice. 2022;**10**(3):1-15. DOI: 10.9745/GHSP-D-21-00525

[29] UN/DESAPD. World Family Planning 2020 Highlights: Accelerating action to ensure universal access to family planning. New York, 10017, USA: United Nations; 2020

[30] Schwandt HM, Speizer IS, Corroon M. Contraceptive service

provider imposed restrictions to contraceptive access in urban Nigeria. BMC Health Services Research. 2017;**17**(1):1-9

[31] Korachais C, Macouillard E, Meessen B. How user fees influence contraception in low and middle income countries: A systematic review. Studies in Family Planning. 2016;**47**(4):341-356

[32] Sacks E, Finlayson K, Brizuela V, Crossland N, Ziegler D, Sauvé C, et al. Factors that influence uptake of routine postnatal care: Findings on women's perspectives from a qualitative evidence synthesis. PLoS One. 2022;**17**(8):e0270264

[33] Sacks E, Langlois ÉV. Postnatal care: Increasing coverage, equity, and quality. The Lancet Global Health. 2016;**4**(7):e442-e443

[34] Wickramasinghe SA, Gunathunga MW, Hemachandra DKNN. Client perceived quality of the postnatal care provided by public sector specialized care institutions following a normal vaginal delivery in Sri Lanka: A cross sectional study. BMC Pregnancy and Childbirth. 2019;**19**(1):1-10

[35] Al-Nakeeb I, Bawazir A, Hattab A. Preventing Adverse Maternal and Perinatal Events from Obstetric Interventions Given Women at Childbirth in Al-Sadaka Teaching Hospital. Aden, Yemen;

[36] Hunker DF, Patrick TE, Albrecht SA, Wisner KL. Is difficult childbirth related to postpartum maternal outcomes in the early postpartum period? Archives of Women's Mental Health. 2009;**12**(4):211-219

[37] Hüner B, Derksen C, Schmiedhofer M, Lippke S, Janni W, Scholz C. Preventable adverse events in obstetrics—systemic assessment of their incidence and linked risk factors. Healthcare. 2022;**2022**:97

[38] Skoogh A, Hall-Lord ML, Bååth C, Bojö A-KS. Adverse events in women giving birth in a labor ward: A retrospective record review study. BMC Health Services Research. 2021;**21**(1):1-8

[39] Ugboaja JO, Berthrand NO, Igwegbe AO, Obi-Nwosu AL. Barriers to postnatal care and exclusive breastfeeding among urbanwomen in southeastern Nigeria. Nigerian Medical Journal: Journal of the Nigeria Medical Association. 2013;**54**(1):45

[40] Balde MD, Diallo A, Soumah AM, Barry F, Touré AO, Camara S. Barriers to utilization of postnatal care: A qualitative study in Guinea. Open Journal of Obstetrics and Gynecology. 2021;**11**(04):391

[41] DiBari JN, Yu SM, Chao SM, Lu MC. Use of postpartum care: predictors and barriers. Journal of pregnancy. 2014;**2014**:1-8. DOI: 10.1155/2014/530769

[42] Williams P, Murindahabi NK, Butrick E, Nzeyimana D, Sayinzoga F, Ngabo B, et al. Postnatal care in Rwanda: facilitators and barriers to postnatal care attendance and recommendations to improve participation. Journal of Global Health Reports 2019;**3**(1):1-9. DOI: 10.29392/joghr.3.e2019032

[43] Kokab F, Jones E, Goodwin L, Taylor B, Kenyon S. Community midwives views of postnatal care in the UK: A descriptive qualitative study. Midwifery. 2022;**104**:103183

Chapter 4

Breastfeeding by Mothers with Cesarean Section Delivery

Nur Intan Kusuma, Siti Khuzaiyah, Nur Chabibah, Rini Kristiyanti, Suparni Suparni and Lia Dwi Prafitri

Abstract

Cesarean section (C-section) is an alternative to childbirth if a normal delivery cannot be achieved. However, in recent decades, the C-section rate has increased in many countries to become more common than vaginal birth. C-section deliveries are associated with lower rates of early initiation breastfeeding. Delay in early initiation of breastfeeding at C-section delivery is related to separation of mother and baby, reduced ability to breastfeed the baby, decreased acceptance of the baby, and lack of milk supply, which can result in shorter duration of breastfeeding. The results of previous studies showed that there was a negative correlation between delivery by C-section and the implementation of early initiation of breastfeeding. This fact indicates that C-section is one of the obstacles in early breastfeeding. Therefore, health workers need to educate the mothers to encourage them to have a spontaneous delivery if there is no medical indication. Suppose indeed the mother needs a C-section for medical reasons. In that case, healthcare professionals (obstetricians, midwives and nurses) also need to optimize the implementation of early breastfeeding initiation for mothers with C-section so that mothers and babies can still gain the experiences and benefits of early breastfeeding initiation and early bonding to the baby.

Keywords: cesarean section (CS), section caesarean delivery, early initiation of breastfeeding, exclusive breastfeeding, postnatal care

1. Introduction

Cesarean section (C-section) is an intervention to overcome complications in labour by delivering the foetus to the uterine wall through the front abdominal wall. Currently, SC is much more performed because of the very development of the procedure [1]. A C-section must still be understood as an alternative to childbirth if a normal delivery cannot be done. Ninety per cent of the delivery processes are normal, while the rest might have complications. Prioritizing the safety of the mother and baby is essential to address the difficulty during labour process [2]. C-section is also associated with maternal and newborn survival, as it can be a life-saving intervention if appropriately indicated [3]. However, in recent decades, the rate of CS has increased in many countries to become more common than vaginal birth [3, 4].

C-section rates worldwide increased from 6.7% in 1990 to 19.1% in 2014 [5]. The increase in CS in various countries can be seen in the following graph (**Figure 1**).

A recent WHO report showed that C-section deliveries continue to rise worldwide, accounting for more than one-fifth (21%) of all deliveries. This figure is expected to rise further in the future decades, with almost one-third (29%) of all newborns predicted to be delivered *via* C-section by 2030 [4]. The trends (1990–2018) and projections (2030) in global, regional and subregional estimates of C-section rates.

By 2030, the C-section rate will be similar in more and less developed countries 36.6% (95% CI 31.7% to 41.4%) and 36.5% (95% CI 32.7% to 40.3%), respectively (**Figure 2**). The C-section rate in the least developed countries will be 11.8% (95% CI 9.7% to 13.8%). In Africa, the Northern sub-region will increase to 48.1% (95% CI 37.4% to 58.8%) CS rate in 2030, while the Sub-Saharan sub-region will remain at 7.1% (95% CI 6.4% to 7.9%). Eastern and Western Asia will reach the 50% mark by 2030, with C-section rates of 63.4% (95% CI 52.9% to 74.0%) and 50.2% (95% CI 47.4% to 52.9%) respectively. Central Asia, on the other hand, has the lowest prediction in this region with a C-section rate of 13.3% (95% CI 2.0% to 24.6%). According to projections for the Americas, 54.3% (95% CI 48.3% to 60.2%) of women in Latin America and the Caribbean will give birth by C-section in 2030, while Northern America will use C-section at a lower rate of 33.8% (95% CI 22.8% to 44.8%). According to projections for Europe, the highest C-section rates are expected in Southern Europe, at 47% (95% CI 38.8% to 53.3%), while C-section will be used in 27.6% (95% CI 16.2% to 39.1%) of births in Northern Europe, with little change over the next decade. In Australia and New Zealand, the use of C-section will rise to 45% (95% CI 38.1% to 52.0%) by 2030 [6]. In current conditions, C-section delivery is not only used as an emergency delivery but as a choice for mothers to give birth even without labour complications.

The trend of selecting C-section as the birth method chosen by mothers is influenced by several reasons, namely women's intense fear of pain and injuries to the mother and child during labour, unpredictability in vaginal delivery, and favorable attitudes or perceived advantages of C-section [7]. In line with the research of Suwanrath et al., [8] which states the results of a qualitative study of mother's reasons

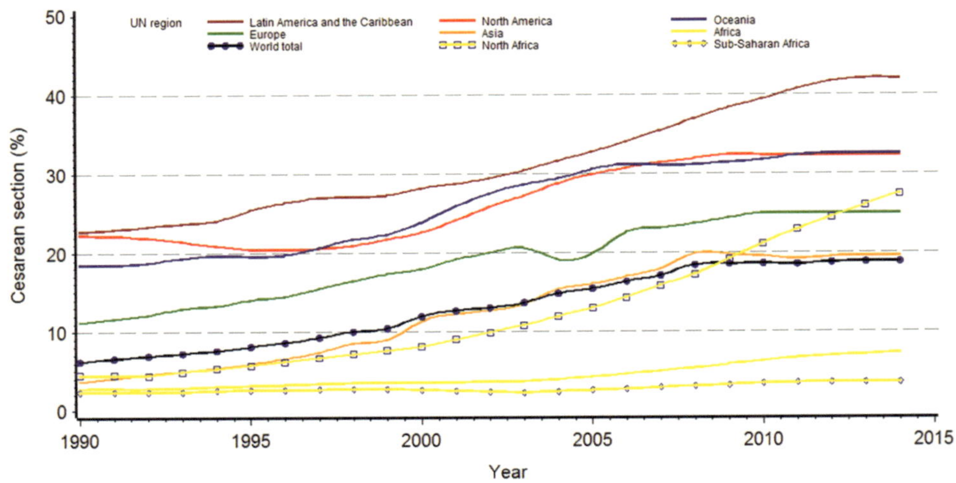

Figure 1.
Global and regional trends in CS, 1990–2014 [5].

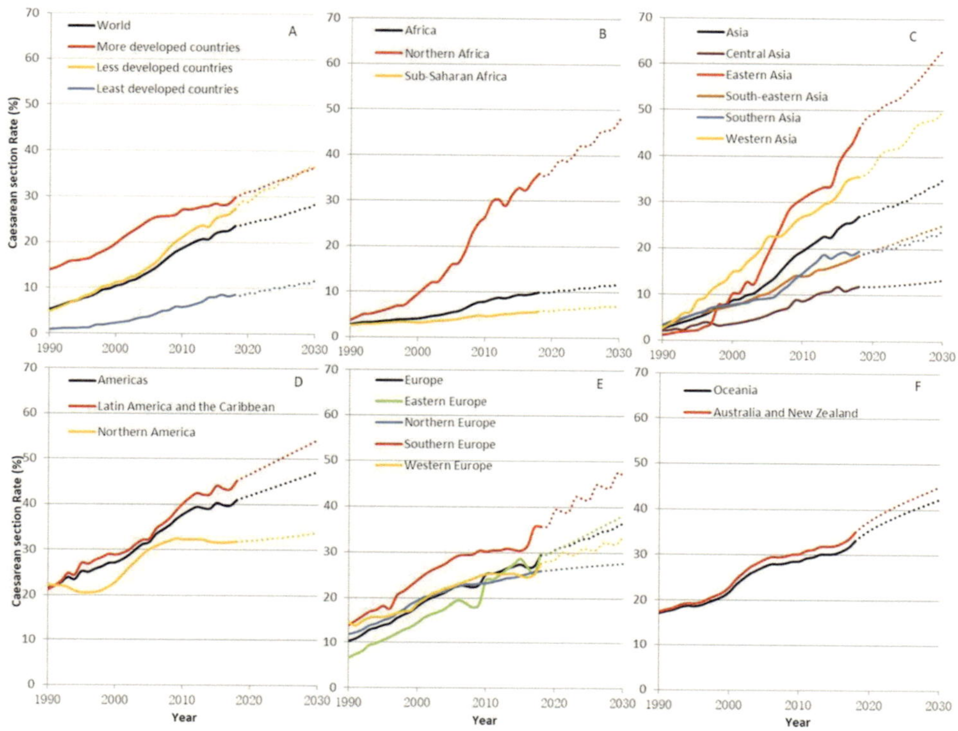

Figure 2.
Trends (1990–2018) and projections (2030) in global, regional and subregional estimates of C-section rates. The solid lines represent trend estimations, while the dotted lines represent predictions. (A) World; (B) Africa; (C) Asia; (D) Americas; (E) Europe; and (F) Oceania. Rates and projections for Melanesia, Micronesia, and Polynesia were not estimated due to the low coverage of data in this Oceania subregion [6].

for C-section preference, such as fear of the birthing process, concerns about safety related to perceived risks that could disrupt health conditions, unpleasant experiences in previous births, positive views towards C-section, access to biased information and belief in auspicious date. Most women choose to give birth by C-section for more than one reason [8]. This increase in C-section delivery occurred globally in both developed and developing countries. This shows that C-section delivery is a global issue that needs special attention and follow-up to reduce it. In addition, this situation must be mindful of because it could have an impact on the health outcomes of mothers and babies.

Recent studies have related C-section delivery with an increased risk of several outcomes later in life, such as type 1 diabetes, asthma and obesity. Another study also stated that mothers who gave birth by C-section were less likely to breastfeed or to delay early initiation of breastfeeding [9]. In fact, early initiation of breastfeeding is one of the keys to the success of exclusive breastfeeding. In addition, early initiation of breastfeeding is important because it has many benefits, namely, it allows the release of colostrum as the baby's first immunity, contains many vitamins and other protective factors, can increase the bond between mother and baby and reduce the risk of postpartum hemorrhage [10]. Delay in early initiation of breastfeeding at C-section is associated with separation of mother and baby, reduced ability to breastfeed the baby, decreased acceptance of the baby, and lack of milk supply, which can result in shorter duration of breastfeeding [9]. The results of previous studies showed that there was a negative correlation between delivery by C-section and the implementation of early initiation of breastfeeding [11]. This shows that C-section is one of the obstacles in early breastfeeding [12]. Therefore, health workers need to provide education to mothers and families if they can give birth spontaneously and do not have medical indications, then delivery can be done spontaneously. If indeed the mother needs a C-section delivery for medical reasons, healthcare professionals (obstetricians, midwives and nurses) also need to optimize the implementation of early initiation of breastfeeding for mothers with C-section delivery so that mothers and babies can still gain the experience of early initiation of breastfeeding and early bonding to the baby [9, 11]. According to the research, a variety of variables, including breastfeeding constraints brought on by the mother's physical discomfort and surgical incision pain, may impair breastfeeding following a C-section. Another study revealed that women who received C-sections experienced breastfeeding challenges. It was discovered through semi-structured interviews that the majority of the mothers had post-C-section nausea, vomiting, and exhaustion. In addition, these women's early postpartum limb numbness from the local anesthetic used during surgery limited their ability to move around and made it more difficult for them to interact with their infants. The majority of women frequently express breastfeeding issues, which are significantly influenced by incision discomfort. Most mothers who undergo a C-section in a South African exploratory study stated that the soreness following the procedure was excruciating [13].

2. The importance of early breastfeeding initiation and breastfeeding practice

Breastfeeding has been recognized as the most effective means of ensuring the health and survival of children. Breastfeeding for the first 6 months is crucial, so the World Health Organization (WHO) recommends related to breastfeeding, such as:

a. Initiate early breastfeeding in the first hour

b. Babies must be exclusively breastfed for 6 months to achieve optimal growth

c. Fulfillment of nutrition for children by providing appropriate and safe complementary foods for babies after 6 months while continuing to be breastfed.

d. Breastfeeding should continue for up to 2 years or beyond [10].

Early Breastfeeding Initiation is the process of giving breast milk to the mother to the baby within the first hour of birth. This is also a step towards ensuring the newborn receives colostrum [14, 15]. Early breastfeeding initiation benefits infants by providing newborn protection from infection and reducing newborn mortality [16]. This process also facilitates the emotional bond between mother and baby which has a positive impact on the duration of exclusive breastfeeding [17]. A mother who starts breastfeeding within an hour of giving birth will stimulate milk production. The milk produced in the first few days is yellow, called colostrum, a vital source of nutrition and immune protection for newborns [10].

In addition to providing protective benefits for the baby, early initiation of breastfeeding also provides an opportunity for skin-to-skin contact (SSC) between mother and baby. Skin-to-skin contact is defined as the practice of laying the baby on the mother's bare chest after the baby is dried and covered with a warm blanket and left for 1 hour after birth [18]. This contact stimulates the release of oxytocin in both mother and baby so it is associated with calm, bonding and reduction of stress, anxiety, and psychological distress [19, 20]. Full-body contact and the sound of a mother's heartbeat are thought to simulate the sensations a baby experiences before birth, further reducing stress. SSC has many benefits for postnatal neuro-physical adjustment [21]. Previous studies have shown that newborns who experience SSC with their mothers have better and more stable physiological functions than newborns who do not have SSC. This is related to newborns' temperature regulation, heart rate, respiration, and gastrointestinal adaption. Babies who experience SSC sleep better, cry less and have fewer painful reactions to routine hospital procedures [21, 22]. This is an important reason for early initiation of breastfeeding after delivery.

The implementation of early breastfeeding initiation is associated with success in continuing exclusive breastfeeding and beyond. Breastfeeding provides health benefits for children and mothers. The benefits of breastfeeding for mothers include helping to accelerate the postpartum involution process thereby reducing the risk of bleeding, reducing stress and accelerating the return of pre-pregnancy weight. Long-term benefits that can be obtained by breastfeeding mothers include reducing the risk of cardiovascular disease, type 2 diabetes, the risk of breast, ovarian and endometrial cancer [23, 24]. In addition to the benefits that mothers get, breastfeeding babies also provides benefits for optimal baby growth and development [25]. Breastfeeding also reduces the risk of infectious diseases in infancy but also reduces the risk of childhood obesity and later metabolic diseases [17, 26].

Exclusive breastfeeding is giving only breast milk for 6 months without any additional food and drinks [27]. However, globally the coverage of exclusive breastfeeding in infants still reaches 44% [28]. UNICEF global databases showed that South Asia achieved the highest exclusive breastfeeding coverage of 61%. Exclusive breastfeeding coverage Eastern and Southern Africa 55%, Latin America and the Caribbean 43%. Eastern Europe, Central Asia, East Asia and the Pacific are at 42% exclusive breastfeeding coverage. Meanwhile, in the West and Central Africa region it was at 38%, then the lowest was in the Middle East and North Africa at 32% [29]. Evidence from research results showed that breastfeeding practice is affected by a variety of sociodemographic (i.e., mother's age, marital status, level of education, employment status, income) and perinatal factors (i.e., parity, method of childbirth, early SSC practice, early initiation of breastfeeding, prenatal class, rooming-in practice) [17]. These factors can be optimized to become reinforcing factors to enable mothers to breastfeed from the first hour after birth.

The evidence about the risks of not breastfeeding for mothers and infants showed that non-breastfed newborns have a higher risk of infectious morbidities, such as an increased risk of childhood obesity, type 1 and type 2 diabetes, leukemia and sudden infant death syndrome (SIDS). Premature infants who are not breastfed are related to a higher risk of necrotizing enterocolitis (NEC). For mothers, failure to breastfeed has been linked with an increased prevalence of premenopausal breast cancer, ovarian cancer, persistent pregnancy weight gain, type 2 diabetes, and metabolic syndrome [30]. Psychologically, mothers who do not breastfeed their babies are reported to experience frustration and feel guilty due to not being able to breastfeed. They think they are not capable of breastfeeding, especially when the baby is crying [31]. This evidence shows that breastfeeding is important in the first hour after birth and continues for 6 months exclusively.

3. The early initiation of breastfeeding and breastfeeding practice by mothers with C-section delivery

Several studies have shown the low practice of early initiation of breastfeeding and breastfeeding in mothers who give birth with C-section delivery [9, 11, 32–36]. In comparison to women who gave birth vaginally, mothers who underwent a C-section had reduced odds of timely initiation of breastfeeding (TIBF), according to the findings of a systematic review. This situation also occurs in studies conducted in Ethiopia, Nigeria, Turkey, Saudi Arabia, Lebanon, Brazil, and India [31]. Another study using data from the Ethiopian Demographic and Health Survey revealed that among mothers who had given birth to their last living child, the prevalence of delayed breastfeeding was 25.03% (95%CI, 20.5–32.2). C-section delivery was one of the important variables linked with delayed breastfeeding initiation [AOR = 4.06 (95%CI, 2.66–6.2)]. The likelihood of delayed initiation of breastfeeding is four times higher among women who had C-section deliveries as compared to women who delivered vaginally [11].

According to a study conducted in Alberta, Canada, more mothers who had planned C-sections had no intention of breastfeeding or did not initiate breastfeeding (7.4% and 4.3%, respectively) than mothers who had a vaginal delivery (3.4% and 1.8%, respectively) or emergency C-sections (2.7% and 2.5%, respectively) [9]. It is also supported by another study that women with vaginal birth are 4.57 (3.16, 6.61) compared to planned C-section deliveries 1.64 (1.09, 2.46) four times more likely to initiate early breastfeeding [37]. According to a meta-analysis of 17 research, the pooled estimate of timely breastfeeding initiation among C-section women in Ethiopia was 40.1% (95% CI 33.29, 46.92). When compared to vaginal birth, C-section was related to a 79% reduced chances of timely breastfeeding initiation (OR 0.21; 95% CI 0.16, 0.28) [38].

According to numerous research, C-section births are related to delays in breastfeeding initiation or perhaps no breastfeeding initiation at all. The duration of breastfeeding in the months that follow may be impacted by this condition. According to the study, women who underwent C-section deliveries had lower rates of both exclusive and general breastfeeding than women who gave birth vaginally. Additionally, consuming formula in the hospital and a delayed start to breastfeeding were associated with C-section birth. The duration of breastfeeding was also reduced after C-section birth (hazard ratio = 1.40, 95% confidence range [1.06, 1.84]) [32]. Another study also showed that Women who had a planned C-section were more likely (OR = 1.61; 95% CI: 1.14, 2.26; p = 0.014) to cease breastfeeding before 12 weeks [9]. Several of these studies show that the practice of early initiation of breastfeeding and breastfeeding by mothers with C-section delivery is still low. The strategy is needed to be able to improve the implementation of early breastfeeding initiation and breastfeeding practices in mothers who deliver by C-section.

4. The barriers in breastfeeding by mothers with C-section Delivery

4.1 Mother's condition after C-section

Based on the literature, several barriers are evident for mothers to make initial contact with the baby, namely the physical condition of the mother including labour pain and limited movement [39, 40]. It was found that most of the mothers experienced nausea, vomiting, and fatigue C-section. Moreover, mothers in the early post-C-section experience numbness of the limbs due to local anesthesia during surgery, experience limitations in physical activity, and have difficulty interacting with newborns. Most mothers stated that pain at the incision was a significant factor for mothers having difficulty breastfeeding [39, 41]. Another study found that the mothers who gave birth by C-section frequently have obstetric-related health issues such as general anesthesia effect, pain, and exhaustion, which delay mother-baby contact [31]. In an exploratory study in South Africa, most mothers stated unbearable pain after C-section. However, some said the pain after a C-section was tolerable and worthwhile [40].

In addition to physical problems, after C-section mothers also experience barriers in psychological conditions. Some literature shows that mothers feel unable to breastfeed because of the baby's condition, the mother's perception that breast milk is insufficient, decreased mother's confidence to breastfeed and uncomfortable position to breastfeed [39–42]. This is in line with a study conducted by Hobbs et al., [9] which found that 62% (n = 1832) of mothers stated that they had more than one difficulty breastfeeding. Studies showed a significant difference between mode of delivery and breastfeeding difficulties with the baby (e.g., latching or sleepy baby), discomfort during breastfeeding (e.g., sore nipples, swollen breasts), and other difficulties (e.g., low milk supply or problems with flat or inverted nipples) [9].

In line with the study conducted on women who underwent a C-Section between July to September 2019 in a Women and Children's Hospital in China showed the results that only six participants (31.58%) chose to exclusively breastfeed, half of all participants used a mix of breast and formula feeding, and three (15.79%) selected formula feeding only. The participants stated that they made the decision to either cease breastfeeding or not to breastfeed because they thought there wasn't enough breast milk to suit their infants' demands. The participants believed that women after C-section have insufficient milk, and therefore, could not start to breastfeed right away [42]. As shown in the literature, mothers often experience frustration and failure due to not being able to breastfeed. They think they are not capable of breastfeeding, especially when the baby is crying. For instance, the mother's belief that her breast milk is insufficient is a significant factor hindering exclusive breastfeeding in China. In addition, mothers said that their infants were sleepy, had trouble sucking on milk, and occasionally even threw up, which frequently caused them to feel frightened and anxious. Thus, mothers' perceptions of infant health affect their breastfeeding practice. For example, it was reported by another study that a mother's perception of baby size might cause delayed breastfeeding in Nicaragua [13].

4.2 Lack of support

The literature showed that mothers with C-sections report a lack of support from health workers in the breastfeeding process. In previous studies, it has been stated repeatedly about the lack of support and patience of family members. In the UK it was reported that mothers felt tired and were not motivated to continue breastfeeding because the family did not support the breastfeeding program. Likewise, women in Hong Kong who do not receive support from their families tend to use formula milk [13]. Supported by another study, the results showed that all mothers had good knowledge about breastfeeding, 26.4% of whom had prior experience in giving breast milk, but only 6.9% and a total of 29.2% started breastfeeding on the first and second day after C-section. Support from health workers in terms of assisting the process of breastfeeding is reported to be low. The correlation test found that the support of health care professionals and the conditions of rooming-in were factors related to the breastfeeding practice (p-value 0.39; p = 0.001; phi value = 0.47; p = 0.001). The low breastfeeding for mothers after C-section correlates with the low support of health care professionals and delays in rooming-in [33].

5. The facilitators to optimize breastfeeding by mothers with C-section Delivery

5.1 Optimizing promotion of breastfeeding during antenatal care

Health services for pregnant women are continuous with delivery, postpartum and newborn health services. Through antenatal care (ANC), promotion and education related to breastfeeding can be conveyed to mothers and their families. Education that needs to be conveyed includes the importance of breastfeeding, the implementation of early initiation breastfeeding and early contact, the right technique to breastfeed, to maintaining breastfeeding until the child is 2 years old can be given to mothers. This aims to prepare pregnant women so they have good knowledge regarding breastfeeding, readiness to breastfeed and self-efficacy for being able to breastfeed after birth [43]. Previous studies suggest that women who learn breastfeeding techniques and have high breastfeeding self-efficacy are more likely to be successful in breastfeeding their babies [44]. Enhancing and investing in healthcare facility ability to facilitate breastfeeding with continuity from prenatal care, early initiation breastfeeding advice, follow-up until hospital discharge, and postpartum care visits might improve exclusive breastfeeding [35].

5.2 Education on normal childbirth for mothers without complications

One of the main goals of every medical team dealing with childbirth is to have a safe delivery [3]. In accordance with the competence of midwives in facilitating clean, safe deliveries and providing a positive experience of the delivery process [45]. C-section was initially introduced to save the condition of the mother and fetus who were in an emergency. However, currently, there is a paradigm shift that C-section is considered an escape from labour pain. In addition, women also have the wrong assumption that C-section is considered painless, safer and healthier than vaginal delivery. In fact, more than half of women voluntarily choose C-section as the preferred mode of delivery [3]. Health education about normal delivery is important and crucial for health workers to restore the perception in women that normal delivery is a physiological process and has less risk than C-section delivery. Women need to be educated that C-sections are only performed in emergency situations in an effort to save the mother and baby. A cross-sectional study among 150 women in India showed that the most common reason for a voluntary C-section was a previous one, which happened 29 times (33%). Besides these, fetal distress (17%), mal-presentations (13%), and maternal request (9%), there were other signs. Most emergency C-sections were done because the baby was in fetal distress (39, or 62%), or because the woman had C-section history in previous labour (12, or 19%) [46]. Another study said that the indication of C-section could come from maternal side, uterine/anatomic side and from fetal side [1].

According to a Norwegian study, primiparous women, those who have had several pregnancies, CS in the past, are older, have a higher gestational age, and have health issues related to pregnancy are less likely to deliver vaginally (gestational diabetes, low-lying placenta, high blood pressure). A model of care with a more natural birth philosophy, not restricting the woman's freedom of movement and position throughout labour and delivery, and continuity of care providers during labour are a few factors that can increase the likelihood of having a normal birth [47]. Raising knowledge of this link and including mothers in decision-making are crucial steps in achieving normal birth [13]. Promotion of normal delivery is achieved with a personalized strategy, encouraging the mother about her capacity, strength and confidence that the mother has to face the normal delivery process. It is important for the mother to feel empowered in the face of labour so that she can achieve a normal delivery and a positive birth experience [48]. Awareness of the mother's ability in the delivery process is expected to increase the mother's self-confidence to undergo a normal delivery process and not choose C-section delivery.

5.3 Policy for implementing C-section delivery procedures according to indications

Taking into account the trend of cases of C-section deliveries that continue to increase, the current policy of C-section deliveries at health care providers needs to be reviewed. The factors that influence the increase in C-section deliveries need to be re-examined to reduce unnecessary C-sections. Health care professionals really need to make strict policies on the implementation of C-section deliveries. This procedure is done if it is to save the mother and baby. It is only recommended when the life of the mother or fetus is threatened [3]. If the mothers do not experience any complications at the end of the pregnancy, C-sections should not be implemented for them [5]. It should be made apparent that a C-section will actually cause complications for the mother and baby.

5.4 Facilitating the mothers with C-sections for early initiation of breastfeeding

Likewise, mothers who give birth vaginally, mothers with C-section delivery also need early contact and early initiation of breastfeeding. A study of women planning an elective C-section birth at a public hospital in New South Wales, Australia found that mothers who had skin-to-skin contact (SSC) during a C-section had positive experiences with better bonding. Mothers also reported lower anxiety and depression than prior C-sections. Chi-square analysis in the intervention group also showed that there was a significant relationship between having SSC and exclusive breastfeeding, $p < 0.005$. According to the odds ratio, newborns ($n = 51$) were twice (OR: 2.24; 95% CI 1.79–2.82) more likely to breastfeed exclusively if they were in the intervention group. A recent study provides evidence of the benefits of skin-to-skin contact during C-section [49].

Studies have shown that skin-to-skin contact after birth enhances innate behavior and the release of maternal oxytocin and can benefit breastfeeding outcomes and early attachment of the mother's baby. Although obstacles were found associated with skin-to-skin contact during C-section. This can be overcome by educating operating room staff about the benefits of SSC so that it can facilitate mothers and babies to do SSC and early initiation of breastfeeding. That study confirms previous findings that new mothers need skilled support and accompaniment after birth [39].

According to the findings of a different study, mothers who underwent an emergency C-section were more likely to have tried breastfeeding their child unsuccessfully before, be unable to do so for the first 24 hours after giving birth, and be unable to do so after leaving the hospital. This is consistent with recent research that found that mothers who gave birth through emergency C-section had a higher likelihood of being unable to breastfeed their child at either the time of delivery or upon discharge. It has been established that early postpartum breastfeeding difficulties and early discontinuation may be related to the mother and fetal stress response associated with delivery issues, particularly those related to C-section. Abdominal surgery's insult in both intended and emergency C-section may equally affect the lacto genesis process, although the notion of an emergency may invoke a greater or prolonged maternal stress response [9]. In these emergency conditions, facilitation for contact as early as possible between mother and baby still needs to be pursued while still paying attention to the condition of the mother and baby.

Research by Zavala-Soto et al. by observing mothers giving birth with C-section who had SSC showed satisfaction felt by the mother, exclusive breastfeeding and continued breastfeeding. The majority of participants in this study group were considered high risk due to previous C-section (39%), abnormal presentation, twins or premature babies, exacerbated diseases such as hypertension and diabetes, or complications during labour (42%). Nevertheless, since the mother's and infant's condition were stable, a pro-breastfeeding C-section was conducted, which included emotional and physical support, a warm environment, woman-centred care and skin-to-skin contact, particularly without interruption with supervised initial feeding at the breast. It was observed that the majority of these women exclusively breastfed for 6 months, including twins and six of eight premature babies (75%) [50]. This shows that optimal facilitation by health care professionals in women giving birth with C-sections can help implement SSC and increase the achievement of exclusive breastfeeding and the continuation of breastfeeding.

5.5 Support of health care professionals, husband and family and community

When mothers are supported at the institution, in the community, or in their families, breastfeeding practices have been found to improve [12, 14, 15].

Offering breastfeeding assistance to women was linked to a 12% lower risk of discontinuing exclusive breastfeeding before the age of 6 months, according to a Cochrane analysis (RR 0.88, 95% CI 0.85–0.92, 46 studies) [14]. Another study discovered that the most successful intervention to increase breastfeeding rates was hospital support that was Baby Friendly Hospital Initiative (BFI), which was linked to a 49% increase in exclusive breastfeeding (RR 1.49, 95% CI 1.33–1.68) and a 20% increase in early breastfeeding initiation (RR 1.20, 95% CI 1.11–1.28) [35]. In line with other study showed that several participants stated that they received positive support from the midwife, especially regarding their breastfeeding problems. The participants felt empowered and developed better relationships with their babies because of the support they received [40].

Difficulties encountered in the early stages of breastfeeding could lead to misperceptions about inadequate milk secretion [13]. This perception can affect the success of breastfeeding postpartum mothers in the future. The comfort of breastfeeding is one of the important factors in stimulating milk secretion, which is a reflex elicited by the baby's sucking. This type of suction can stimulate the secretion of prolactin which is secreted from the anterior lobe of the pituitary gland. However, the pain from a C-section and anxiety suppresses both prolactin and milk secretion because pain stimulates the release of catecholamine neurotransmitters. The results of previous studies show that 2–5 days after delivery, the secretion of breast milk in women with C-sections is less than in women with vaginal birth. Furthermore, psychological adjustment after C-section interferes with the mother's learning about maternal and infant care skills and makes her feel incompetent in breastfeeding [13]. Therefore, C-section is a significant obstacle to early initiation of breastfeeding [51]. This condition indicates that mothers with C-sections really need support to be able to breastfeed their babies. There is evidence to suggest that professional support or the support of trained and experienced health workers supports the continuation of breastfeeding [35]. Women undergoing C-section need more specialized resources that can provide mental and physical support for breastfeeding, especially in the early postpartum period. It is also critical to promote optimal postpartum nursing positions, such as "biological nurturing." Breast milk volume and maternal self-efficacy could be improved by maintaining a comfortable breastfeeding position and hastening postoperative recovery [42].

5.6 Implementing breastfeeding support

WHO has provided guidance on 'Counseling women to improve breastfeeding practice', which was compiled based on a systematic literature review and developed by a group of international experts. The policy expands on prior recommendations from the 'Global Strategy for Infant and Young Child Feeding' and increases the strength of the recommendation for breastfeeding counseling. It provides evidence-based breastfeeding counseling suggestions: (1) Every pregnant woman and mother with newborns or young children should get breastfeeding counseling. (2) Breastfeeding counseling should be provided during both the antenatal and postnatal periods, for a duration of up to 24 months or longer. (3) Breastfeeding counseling should be offered at least six times and as required. (4) Face-to-face breastfeeding counseling should be provided. Breastfeeding counseling may also be delivered over the phone or through other remote ways of counseling. (5) Breastfeeding counseling should be offered as part of a continuum of care by suitably qualified healthcare professionals as well as community-based lay and peer breastfeeding counselors. and (6) Breastfeeding counseling should anticipate and overcome major breastfeeding issues and situations, as well as help the mothers to develop skills, competencies and confidence. By implementing breastfeeding counseling optimally for mothers and families, it is hoped that it can increase the understanding of mothers and families and increase the self-efficacy of mothers to breastfeed their babies [52].

6. Conclusion

Cesarean Section (C-section) delivery is a global issue in maternal and child health care. Mothers who gave birth by C-section could have an impact on delays in SSC and early initiation of breastfeeding. This in turn can lead to a shorter duration of breastfeeding and hinder the attainment of exclusive breastfeeding. C-section deliveries without indications should not be performed on the mother. This method is only performed on mothers or babies with emergency conditions. Mothers who give birth by C-sections still need to be facilitated for initial contact and early initiation of breastfeeding for their babies so that bonding can be established between mother and baby. Assistance in overcoming breastfeeding difficulties is carried out with the help and support of health workers, families and the community. Healthcare professionals are really expected to be able to provide education and facilitate mothers with C-sections to maintain early skin-to-skin contact in the context of early initiation of breastfeeding and as an effort to increase the duration of breastfeeding in mothers with C-sections delivery. It is also important to provide breastfeeding promotion and education to mothers and their families so that they have an adequate understanding of breastfeeding, even for mothers with C-sections.

Conflict of interest

The authors declare no conflict of interest.

Author details

Nur Intan Kusuma*, Siti Khuzaiyah, Nur Chabibah, Rini Kristiyanti, Suparni Suparni and Lia Dwi Prafitri
Universitas Muhammadiyah Pekajangan Pekalongan, Indonesia

*Address all correspondence to: intan@umpp.ac.id; intankusuma29@gmail.com

IntechOpen

© 2023 The Author(s). Licensee IntechOpen. This chapter is distributed under the terms of the Creative Commons Attribution License (http://creativecommons.org/licenses/by/3.0), which permits unrestricted use, distribution, and reproduction in any medium, provided the original work is properly cited.

References

[1] Sung S, Mahdy H. Cesarean Section. Treasure Island (FL): StatPearls Publishing; 2022

[2] Hofmeyr GJ, Barrett JF, Crowther CA. Planned caesarean section for women with a twin pregnancy. Cochrane Database of Systematic Reviews. 2015;**12**:CD006553. pub2. DOI: 10.1002/14651858.CD006553.pub2

[3] Zakerihamidi M, Roudsari RL, Merghati E. Vaginal delivery vs. Cesarean section: A focused ethnographic study of Women's perceptions in the north of Iran. International Journal of Community Based Nursing and Midwifery. 2015;**3**:39-50

[4] World Health Organization. Caesarean Section Rates Continue to Rise, Amid Growing Inequalities in Access 2021. Available from: https://www.who.int/news/item/16-06-2021-caesarean-section-rates-continue-to-rise-amid-growing-inequalities-in-access [Accessed: December 21, 2022]

[5] Betrán AP, Ye J, Moller A-B, Zhang J, Gülmezoglu AM, Torloni MR. The increasing trend in caesarean section rates: Global, regional and National Estimates: 1990-2014. PLoS One. 2016;**11**:e0148343. DOI: 10.1371/journal.pone.0148343

[6] Betran AP, Ye J, Moller A-B, Souza JP, Zhang J. Trends and projections of caesarean section rates: Global and regional estimates. BMJ Global Health. 2021;**6**:e005671. DOI: 10.1136/bmjgh-2021-005671

[7] Colomar M, Opiyo N, Kingdon C, Long Q, Nion S, Bohren MA, et al. Do women prefer caesarean sections? A qualitative evidence synthesis of their views and experiences. PLoS One. 2021;**16**:e0251072. DOI: 10.1371/journal.pone.0251072

[8] Suwanrath C, Chunuan S, Matemanosak P, Pinjaroen S. Why do pregnant women prefer cesarean birth? A qualitative study in a tertiary care center in southern Thailand. BMC Pregnancy and Childbirth. 2021;**21**:23. DOI: 10.1186/s12884-020-03525-3

[9] Hobbs AJ, Mannion CA, McDonald SW, Brockway M, Tough SC. The impact of caesarean section on breastfeeding initiation, duration and difficulties in the first four months postpartum. BMC Pregnancy and Childbirth. 2016;**16**:90. DOI: 10.1186/s12884-016-0876-1

[10] World Health Organization. Breastfeeding 2018. Available from: https://www.who.int/news-room/facts-in-pictures/detail/breastfeeding [Accessed: December 9, 2022].

[11] Gedefaw G, Goedert MH, Abebe E, Demis A. Effect of cesarean section on initiation of breast feeding: Findings from 2016 Ethiopian demographic and health survey. PLoS One. 2020;**15**:e0244229. DOI: 10.1371/journal.pone.0244229

[12] Johar N, Mohamad N, Saddki N, Tengku Ismail TA, Sulaiman Z. Factors associated with early breastfeeding initiation among women who underwent Cesarean Delivery at tertiary hospitals in Kelantan, Malaysia. Korean Journal of Family Medicine. 2021;**42**:140-149. DOI: 10.4082/kjfm.19.0178

[13] Li L, Wan W, Zhu C. Breastfeeding after a cesarean section: A literature review. Midwifery. 2021;**103**:103117. DOI: 10.1016/j.midw.2021.103117

[14] Mary JJF, Sindhuri R, Kumaran AA, Dongre AR. Early initiation of breastfeeding and factors associated with its delay among mothers at discharge from a single hospital. Clinical and Experimental Pediatrics. 2022;**65**:201-208. DOI: 10.3345/cep.2021.00129

[15] Ekubay M, Berhe A, Yisma E. Initiation of breastfeeding within one hour of birth among mothers with infants younger than or equal to 6 months of age attending public health institutions in Addis Ababa, Ethiopia. International Breastfeeding Journal. 2018;**13**:4. DOI: 10.1186/s13006-018-0146-0

[16] Berkat S, Sutan R. The effect of early initiation of breastfeeding on neonatal mortality among low birth weight in Aceh Province, Indonesia: An unmatched case control study. Advances in Epidemiology. 2014;**2014**:1-7. DOI: 10.1155/2014/358692

[17] Cozma-Petruţ A, Filip L, Banc R, Mîrza O, Gavrilaş L, Ciobârcă D, et al. Breastfeeding practices and determinant factors of exclusive breastfeeding among mothers of children aged 0-23 months in northwestern Romania. Nutrients. 2021;**13**:3998. DOI: 10.3390/nu13113998

[18] UNICEF. Skin-to-Skin Contact. Baby Friendly Initiative 2022. Available from: https://www.unicef.org.uk/babyfriendly/baby-friendly-resources/implementing-standards-resources/skin-to-skin-contact/ [Accessed: December 23, 2022]

[19] Ionio C, Ciuffo G, Landoni M. Parent–infant skin-to-skin contact and stress regulation: A systematic review of the literature. International Journal of Environmental Research and Public Health. 2021;**18**:4695. DOI: 10.3390/ijerph18094695

[20] Krol KM, Grossmann T. Psychological effects of breastfeeding on children and mothers. Bundesgesundheitsbl. 2018;**61**:977-985. DOI: 10.1007/s00103-018-2769-0

[21] Bigelow AE, Power M. Mother–infant skin-to-skin contact: Short- and long-term effects for mothers and their children born full-term. Frontiers in Psychology. 2020;**11**:1921. DOI: 10.3389/fpsyg.2020.01921

[22] Widström A, Brimdyr K, Svensson K, Cadwell K, Nissen E. Skin-to-skin contact the first hour after birth, underlying implications and clinical practice. Acta Paediatrica. 2019;**108**:1192-1204. DOI: 10.1111/apa.14754

[23] Dieterich CM, Felice JP, O'Sullivan E, Rasmussen KM. Breastfeeding and health outcomes for the mother-infant dyad. Pediatric Clinics of North America. 2013;**60**:31-48. DOI: 10.1016/j.pcl.2012.09.010

[24] Doan TTD, Binns C, Pham NM, Zhao Y, Dinh TPH, Bui TTH, et al. Improving breastfeeding by empowering mothers in Vietnam: A randomised controlled trial of a Mobile app. International Journal of Environmental Research and Public Health. 2020;**17**:5552. DOI: 10.3390/ijerph17155552

[25] United Nations Children's Fun. UNICEF. Breastfeeding: A Mother's Gift, for Every Child. 2018

[26] The Association of Women's Health, Obstetric and, Neonatal Nurses. Breastfeeding and the Use of Human Milk. Journal of Obstetric, Gynecologic & Neonatal Nursing. 2021;**50**:e1-e5. DOI: 10.1016/j.jogn.2021.06.006

[27] WHO | Breastfeeding. WHO n.d. Available from: http://www.who.int/nutrition/topics/exclusive_breastfeeding/en/ [Accessed: December 21, 2022]

[28] World Health Organization. World Breastfeeding Week 2022. World Health Organization - Regional Office for the Eastern Mediterranean 2022. Available from: http://www.emro.who.int/nutrition/campaigns/world-breastfeeding-week-2022.html [Accessed: December 21, 2022]

[29] UNICEF. Breastfeeding. UNICEF DATA 2022. Available from: https://data.unicef.org/topic/nutrition/breastfeeding/ [Accessed: March 22, 2023]

[30] Stuebe A. The risks of not breastfeeding for mothers and infants. Reviews in Obstetrics & Gynecology. 2009;**2**:222-231. DOI: 10.3909/riog0093

[31] Teshale AB, Tesema GA. Timely initiation of breastfeeding and associated factors among mothers having children less than two years of age in sub-Saharan Africa: A multilevel analysis using recent demographic and health surveys data. PLoS One. 2021;**16**:e0248976. DOI: 10.1371/journal.pone.0248976

[32] Chen C, Yan Y, Gao X, Xiang S, He Q, Zeng G, et al. Influences of Cesarean Delivery on Breastfeeding Practices and Duration: A Prospective Cohort Study. Journal of Human Lactation. 2018;**34**:526-534. DOI: 10.1177/0890334417741434

[33] Wulandari DR, Dewanti L. Rendahnya Praktik Menyusui pada Ibu Post Sectio Caesarea dan Dukungan Tenaga Kesehatan di Rumah Sakit. Kesmas: National Public Health Journal. 2014;**8**:393. DOI: 10.21109/kesmas.v8i8.410

[34] Hunter T, Cattelona G. Breastfeeding initiation and duration in first-time mothers: Exploring the impact of father involvement in the early post-partum period breastfeeding. Health Promotion Perspectives. 2014. DOI: 10.5681/HPP.2014.017

[35] Kinshella M-LW, Salimu S, Vidler M, Banda M, Molyneux EM, Dube Q, et al. Beyond early initiation: A qualitative study on the challenges of hospital-based postpartum breastfeeding support. PLOS Global Public Health. 2022;**2**:e0001266. DOI: 10.1371/journal.pgph.0001266

[36] Hernández-Cordero S, Lozada-Tequeanes AL, Fernández-Gaxiola AC, Shamah-Levy T, Sachse M, Veliz P, et al. Barriers and facilitators to breastfeeding during the immediate and one month postpartum periods, among Mexican women: A mixed methods approach. International Breastfeeding Journal. 2020;**15**:87. DOI: 10.1186/s13006-020-00327-3

[37] Taha Z, Ali Hassan A, Wikkeling-Scott L, Papandreou D. Prevalence and associated factors of caesarean section and its impact on early initiation of breastfeeding in Abu Dhabi, United Arab Emirates. Nutrients. 2019;**11**:2723. DOI: 10.3390/nu11112723

[38] Getaneh T, Negesse A, Dessie G, Desta M, Temesgen H, Getu T, et al. Impact of cesarean section on timely initiation of breastfeeding in Ethiopia: A systematic review and meta-analysis. International Breastfeeding Journal. 2021;**16**:51. DOI: 10.1186/s13006-021-00399-9

[39] Chaplin J, Kelly J, Kildea S. Maternal perceptions of breastfeeding difficulty after caesarean section with regional anaesthesia: A qualitative study. Women and Birth. 2016;**29**:144-152. DOI: 10.1016/j.wombi.2015.09.005

[40] Jikijela TP, James S, Sonti BSI. Caesarean section deliveries: Experiences of mothers of midwifery care at a public hospital in Nelson Mandela Bay. Curationis. 2018;**41**:1-9. DOI: 10.4102/curationis.v41i1.1804

[41] Ouyang Y-Q, Su M, Redding SR. A survey on difficulties and desires of breast-feeding women in Wuhan, China. Midwifery. 2016;**37**:19-24. DOI: 10.1016/j.midw.2016.03.014

[42] Wen J, Yu G, Kong Y, Liu F, Wei H. An exploration of the breastfeeding behaviors of women after cesarean section: A qualitative study. International Journal of Nursing Sciences. 2020;**7**:419-426. DOI: 10.1016/j.ijnss.2020.07.008

[43] Lumbiganon P, Martis R, Laopaiboon M, Festin MR, Ho JJ, Hakimi M. Antenatal breastfeeding education for increasing breastfeeding duration. Cochrane Database of Systematic Reviews. 2016;**2016**:1-79. DOI: 10.1002/14651858.CD006425.pub4

[44] Wu S-FV, Chen S-C, Liu H-Y, Lee H-L, Lin Y-E. Knowledge, intention, and self-efficacy associated with breastfeeding: Impact of these factors on breastfeeding during postpartum hospital stays in Taiwanese women. International Journal of Environmental Research and Public Health. 2021;**18**:5009. DOI: 10.3390/ijerph18095009

[45] World Health Organization. Midwifery Education and Care 2022. Available from: https://www.who.int/teams/maternal-newborn-child-adolescent-health-and-ageing/maternal-health/midwifery [Accessed: December 27, 2022]

[46] Singh N, Pradeep Y, Jauhari S. Indications and determinants of cesarean section: A cross-sectional study. International Journal of Applied and Basic Medical Research. 2020;**10**:280. DOI: 10.4103/ijabmr.IJABMR_3_20

[47] Prosser SJ, Barnett AG, Miller YD. Factors promoting or inhibiting normal birth. BMC Pregnancy and Childbirth. 2018;**18**:241. DOI: 10.1186/s12884-018-1871-5

[48] Dahlberg U, Persen J, Skogås A-K, Selboe S-T, Torvik HM, Aune I. How can midwives promote a normal birth and a positive birth experience? The experience of first-time Norwegian mothers. Sexual & Reproductive Healthcare. 2016;7:2-7. DOI: 10.1016/j.srhc.2015.08.001

[49] Sheedy GM, Stulz VM, Stevens J. Exploring outcomes for women and neonates having skin-to-skin contact during caesarean birth: A quasi-experimental design and qualitative study. Women and Birth. 2022;**35**:e530-e538. DOI: 10.1016/j.wombi.2022.01.008

[50] Zavala-Soto JO, Hernandez-Rivero L, Tapia-Fonllem C. Pro-lactation cesarean section: Immediate skin-to-skin contact and its influence on prolonged breastfeeding. Frontiers in Sociology. 2022;**7**:908811. DOI: 10.3389/fsoc.2022.908811

[51] Lisien C-F, Fu J-C, Long C-Y, Lin H-S. Factors influencing breast symptoms in breastfeeding women after Cesarean section Delivery. Asian Nursing Research. 2011;**5**:88-98. DOI: 10.1016/S1976-1317(11)60017-0

[52] WHO. Guideline: Counselling of Women to Improve Breastfeeding Practices. 2018

Section 3

Postnatal Challenges

Chapter 5

Addressing Postnatal Challenges: Effective Strategies for Postnatal Care

Ejura Ochala

Abstract

Delivery of the placenta marks the end of pregnancy and the beginning of puerperium. Puerperium or postnatal period is a period of transition, it is the extended period between the completion of the third stage of delivery till 42 days (6 weeks) after childbirth. It is a critical time requiring the most attention on the mother, baby, and family members. Many mothers experience near-miss events and maternal and infant deaths occur during this time. However, it is a most overlooked period. Mothers experience numerous changes which include physiological, psychological economic and sociological changes and without the necessary knowledge and support could affect their ability to care for the newborn and themselves. Challenges mothers experience include the decision to breastfeed and care for the baby, medical conditions associated with pregnancy and puerperium, postpartum hemorrhage, preeclampsia, increased cesarean section rate and complications and high delivery cost. International health bodies have recommendations for postnatal care, this chapter will focus on strategies the mothers and care providers can adopt to overcome postnatal challenges.

Keywords: challenges, mothers, postnatal care, postnatal challenges, postpartum strategies

1. Introduction

Pregnancy and its unique processes come with a variety of experiences and emotions. Due to the different physiologic makeup, adaptation, and responses, individual women respond differently to normal pregnancy processes. Women, therefore, need support to navigate the challenges of puerperium. Midwives are uniquely trained, skilled, and placed to meet these needs.

Delivery of the placenta marks the end of pregnancy and the beginning of puerperium. Puerperium or postnatal period is a period of transition, it is the extended period between the completion of the third stage of delivery up till 42 days (6 weeks) after childbirth. It is a critical time requiring the most attention on the mother, baby, and family members. Many mothers experience near-miss events and maternal and infant deaths occur during this time. However, the immediate postpartum period appears to be the most overlooked [1–3].

Challenges mothers experience include the decision to breastfeed and how to care for the baby, medical conditions associated with pregnancy and puerperium, postpartum hemorrhage, preeclampsia, increased cesarean section rate and complications, and high delivery cost. This chapter will provide suggestions for adjusting to the physiologic and psychological changes of pregnancy during puerperium.

2. Postnatal challenges and coping strategies

Mothers experience numerous changes which include physiological, psychological economic, and sociological changes, and without the necessary knowledge and support could affect their ability to care for the newborn and themselves.

2.1 Physiologic challenges

The human body witnesses several physiologic changes during pregnancy, some of which resolve or culminate in other conditions during the puerperium. There are increases in the activity of all organs from the cardiovascular to the respiratory, renal, endocrine, gastrointestinal, skeletal, and integumentary systems. These are characterized by increased cardiac output and heart rate (20–45%), 20% more oxygen demand, about 50% increased renal flow and function, delayed gastric emptying and reduced albumin level, 9–12 kg increase in body weight, relaxation of joints, reduced calcium, increased activity of the skin and mucus membranes [4].

These are normal changes during pregnancy, though may cause discomfort as the pregnancy advances. The woman must seek nursing and medical advice in cases of serious discomfort or interference with normal daily function. The advice comes in handy during antenatal sessions where the mother can ask pertinent questions and get clarifications as well as self-help advice from the midwife.

Physiologic challenges in puerperium may result from the reversal of some of the changes that occurred during pregnancy and cuts across all systems of the body as well. Firstly, the cardiovascular system experiences further increased cardiac volume from the contracting uterus which decreases within 24 hours and gradually returns to pre-pregnancy level in 4–6 weeks. There is increased body temperature from pain, fatigue, and increased blood flow, this also normalizes a few hours after birth. Pain on the episiotomy site and puerperal infection are notable causes of pyrexia [5].

Other physiologic challenges postpartum mothers experience include musculoskeletal disorder and or dysfunction. Pelvic floor dysfunction (PFD) and diastasis recti abdominis (DRA) are associated with pregnancy and childbirth. They have negative effects on the physical, psychological, and social life of the woman [6].

2.2 Psychological challenges

Pregnancy and puerperium come with multiple and numerous challenges for primipara and multiparous women. The task of caring for a new child, breastfeeding and combining it with work and family responsibilities can be enormous for women who are contending with drastic changes in their physics. Every woman responds differently and must develop adaptive skills to navigate these phases of motherhood.

The pregnant woman faces mixed emotional changes and psychological support is important to pull through the mood changes, exhaustion and or alternating elation, and need for affection, sexual. Pregnancy is a stressor to some women; the anxiety and emotional instability can lead to preterm labour and preterm delivery in a quarter to two-thirds of women affected. Therefore, pregnant women require more support from partners and social and medical teams. The absence of psychological support during pregnancy and through the postpartum period could lead to postnatal depression and an inability to cope with childcare, self-care, and independent economic life [7].

Evidence shows adopting a positive psychological attitude during pregnancy supports psychological well-being in the puerperium. Women must develop elevated levels of resilience to cope with the added stress during puerperium for adequate self-care, coping with the infant and other social duties as a wife and mother [8, 9].

Women sometimes experience several negative and positive emotions, anxiety and psychological symptoms during pregnancy which often are associated with hormonal factors and the need for relationships. The emotional instability is more pronounced during the stress of labour, initiating breastfeeding and fitting into the motherhood role postpartum. Measuring into the motherhood role is therefore challenging necessitating the psychological support by the midwife. Midwives must create a tranquil environment to support the mothers' adjustments [10].

2.2.1 Causes of unstable psychological state in the puerperium

Many women are at risk of abnormal psychologic adjustment postnatally. Such women include mothers of babies diagnosed or born with birth defects [11], sociodemographic factors like low-income status, mode of delivery, and cultural practices with a preference for the male child [12], lack of social and psychologic support with bonding failures [13] positive history of prenatal psychologic symptoms and in clients with greater than one psychologic disorder [14] hereditary and family history of mental disorder [15].

Motherhood is a new role and can be challenging for multipara and first-time mothers. Social and societal norms are expected of new mothers. Childbirth is a social phenomenon; some women find it difficult to fit into these roles or function within acclaimed roles [16]. The ineffective social support during pregnancy affects the psychological state of mothers and could lead to failed bonding perinatally [13]. The inability to cope with the stress and challenges of breastfeeding affects mental health and adaptation to the new role. It may also result in delayed lactation, reduce the confidence to conduct breastfeeding and affect the newborn negatively [17].

2.2.2 Signs of altered postpartum psychologic state management

There exists a chasm between actual and perceived altered postpartum psychological state. It is one syndrome that is underreported and undiagnosed due to the level of health provider knowledge, skill and competence stigma attached [18]. Signs of altered psychological state include increased anxiety and fear, and poor maternal-infant bonding, poor maternal health and feeding [19, 20]. Low resilience and high stress perception are also associated with poor psychological coping [9].

Unidentified and untreated psychological concerns can interfere with the successful motherhood experience and social life of the woman [21]. Though midwives can identify and care for women with psychological disorders, they tend to refer such to other professionals. The psychological challenges encountered in puerperium could be managed effectively by maternity nurses [22].

Midwives play significant roles in screening, treating, and referring identified cases for expert management [23]. Other ways of managing postpartum psychologic challenges include hospital/facility-based care [24], and community and out-stationed care where networks and support groups are formed to help such clients [25]. The recent pandemic equally saw the introduction of mobile dyadic clinics to cater to the needs of such clients who would otherwise not assess care due to difficult social situations [26].

Another approach is by giving the client a voice, and an opportunity to express self and be heard. This will improve communication with the caregiver as the woman gains confidence, learns to trust, and relieves anxious feelings [27]. Moreover, providing both antenatal and postnatal counseling with reading/supportive literature, giving physical therapy like massage, and yoga, and through scheduled telephone calls from providers [28].

2.2.3 Importance of psychologic support during the postpartum

A stable maternal psychological state is a pre-requisite for effective coping, midwives must support and design/institute measures to enhance coping and prevent postpartum depression, anxiety, and stress. Some of the measures include providing information, creating opportunities to discuss fears and clarify doubts, and initiating breastfeeding early with support for women who do not lactate early. The midwife must explore the option of getting family presence and social support for women who demand it and for those without family presence.

It is also important to screen postpartum women to identify risk factors for psychological maladjustment and institute measures to mitigate them. There is also

Midwives' intervention	Actions
Informational support	Providing information about the care available through education, explanation, and clarification of doubts
Emotional support	Giving emotional support through verbal encouragement, attentive listening and providing answers to questions Non-verbal care such as touch and hugs to emotionally unstable mothers who consent.
Providing self-care support	Self-care support like doing cord-care, bathing and changing baby's clothes/diapers and feeding the baby
Psychologic assessment and screening	Routinely assess and document the psychological well-being of mothers to provide bases for action
Multisectoral approach	Encourage collaboration and consultation with the interdisciplinary team

Adapted from Sangsawang et al. [29].

Table 1.
Psychological interventions for postpartum women.

a need to encourage disclosures of untoward familial psychological states to enable early comprehensive assessment and treatment. **Table 1** shows some psychological assessments and interventions midwives can give to postpartum women.

2.2.4 Strategies to overcome the postpartum psychological challenge

Midwives contribute to the psychological well-being of new mothers by providing adequate care and partner support during labour and immediate puerperium. Encouraging mind and physical relaxation, early ambulation and exercise, socialization and interaction with family, peers, and colleagues to gain support and overcome stress [30].

Midwives can provide improved rapport and social support during pregnancy and encourage others to do the same. They can introduce the women to support groups online where they can interact and share thoughts as they transit through puerperium [13]. Another approach is to enable midwife-family-mediated support. The midwife here serves as the go-between the woman and her family, providing information and support to the woman and family as well as galvanizing family support for the mother. They also reduce the cost of care by enlightening mothers on how to take advantage of family support [29].

It is not enough to theoretically teach the breastfeeding method. A step further demonstration of breastfeeding interventions will further build their confidence and help mothers internalize the education [17]. A fourth strategy is adopting a systematic approach to the care of postpartum women. Using empathy and love, the wholistic midwifery framework leaves no system out, the mother must be assessed at each contact with the health practitioner, communicating care and providing a prompt referral to a higher level of care once any deviation is envisaged.

Moreover, maintaining standards of care and education of midwives is necessary for rapid identification, diagnosis, and treatment of psychological deviations in postpartum women. Also ensuring all postpartum women have access to follow-up care will enhance their performance of the women [31].

Postnatal care is an aspect of maternal and child health care that appears to have received minimal attention. Midwives, postnatal mothers, and their families tend to disregard postnatal visits, assuming that physical recovery is always guaranteed when a mother has had a normal pregnancy and childbirth. Unfortunately, preventable complications occurred during this period [32]. Encourage and ensure routine postnatal attendance and screening of mothers and their babies.

Other strategies to help women adjust to postnatal challenges include building their capacity through formal education and self-empowerment of midwives and other caregivers.

2.3 Sociologic and economic challenge

Women are revered for their role in procreation, however, different social, psychological, economic, and environmental factors with the status of these women and the demands of pregnancy pose a challenge to them. Pregnancy and the process of childbearing have social implication that affects a woman. The current wave of diseases and social unrest complicates the struggles of pregnant and breastfeeding women, reducing their coping ability and susceptibility to psychological and social stress [33].

Howbeit the presence of strong social and economic support increases the coping capacity of women.

3. The role of the midwife in combating postpartum challenges

The International Confederation of Midwives [34] in a Core document stipulates the functions of a Midwife include safeguarding the health and rights of the mothers and their babies. Midwives support and promote natural birthing without interference. They provide respectful, anticipatory, and adaptable care that takes cognizance of the needs of the woman, her newborn, family, and community. And have the capacity for timely patient referral for appropriate secondary care with appropriate technology. With the additional role of informing and collaborating with others to provide essential care to the woman, her child and the family.

They provide pertinent education to mothers and support the ability to make informed decisions. Midwives empower women to be accountable and responsible for their health and those of their families. Provide improved care and service to the mother, baby, and family through inter and intra-professional collaboration and consultation. They must be accountable for individual and collective advancement of midwifery knowledge and care through involvement in continuing education and mentoring and teaching the future generation of midwives.

Midwives play pivotal roles in the health sector, the system benefits from a midwife-led team. Midwife-led teams promote cohesion and cooperation of members. The approach promotes increased benefits of continuity of care with good fetal and maternal outcomes, which are cost-effective and adaptable. Teamwork is enhanced among health workers and the comradery spirit and autonomy of members are promoted [35].

Professional midwifery practice contributes to a decline in infant and maternal illness and deaths [36, 37]. Improves maternal satisfaction and a willingness to continue in the care continuum [38]. The non-medicalization approach of midwifery care contributes to a reduction in the cost of healthcare across low and high-income nations. Countries can divert such funds to staff training and improvement of service [39].

A midwife (Accoucheuse) assesses and screens clients to identify risks, preventing and instituting early treatment for women at risk of psychological disorders. They also offer culturally sensitive care to women while integrating mental health services into basic maternal healthcare [40]. They give psychosocial support to the woman and relatives, enabling effective coping [29].

The education given during health and postnatal visits helps to empower the woman with information for decision-making, self-reliance, and self-determination [41]. This also improves the women's skills in childcare and breastfeeding [17]. Moreover, midwives support women in achieving their fertility and contraceptive goals using contraceptives and family planning education [42].

Similarly, midwives support women to adopt healthy and healthful futuristic reproductive behaviors [43]. Midwives ensure the safety of women and their babies. They give quality maternal care during safe and unsafe periods, and their life and health are often sacrificed to preserve women and their babies. They identify and provide counseling to women at risk or are victims of intimate partner violence, providing anonymous and confidential treatment to victims [44].

During the postpartum period, it is essential and expected that the woman makes four (4) contacts with the midwife to provide continuous care. Care is divided into three stages: 24 hours after birth, 7 days after delivery and 6 weeks postpartum. However, care in the first 24 hours is critical and lays the foundation for subsequent care. Where the mother cannot make or afford all four meetings, receiving comprehensive midwifery care on the first day is a solid foundation [45].

3.1 Care within 24 hours of birth

3.1.1 First-hour postpartum care

Ensure the safety and comfort of the mother. The midwife must ensure that the woman is clean and comfortable and that all soiled or wet linen is replaced with clean, warm clothing. The delivery suite is tidy, and all sharps are discarded for the safety of patients and staff.

Examine the perineum and assess for damage. If any tear or episiotomy, the midwife must ensure they are promptly sutured, and the woman is educated on how to care for bruises and the suture site, asepsis must be maintained in care of these areas.

Take and record the woman's vital signs including the record of blood loss. This is compared with the vital signs during labour and serves as a baseline for future vital signs reading to identify early deviation from normal.

Assess the woman's physical and physiologic status: the nipple for readiness to breastfeed. An inverted nipple may be detected at this stage, though it might have been identified and care is taken to ensure its prominence.

The midwife must measure the symphysio-fundal height to rule out retained placenta/product or retained twin. Symphysio-fundal height of 22–24 cm or at the level of the umbilicus is normal. It should however decrease by 1 cm daily until it cannot be measured or returned to the pelvic cavity [46].

3.1.2 Skin-to-skin contact

The infant is brought in contact with the mother within one hour of birth to stimulate bonding, initiate early breastfeeding and lactation, overcome breastfeeding barriers, increase the temperature of the baby and ability to overcome the stress of delivery, initiate self-control, and cope with future stress [47].

3.1.3 Care of the child

The newborn is susceptible without skilled midwifery care, preventing and reducing neonatal and infant mortality. The midwife is the surest person to provide the utmost neonatal care for the neonate. The three essential needs of the neonate after establishing respiration are the need for warmth, protection from infection and nutrition. As early and sustained skin-to-skin contact provides warmth, the mother's body temperature helps regulate the neonate's temperature. Bonding begins early, comforting the newborn and initiating breastfeeding [48, 49].

3.1.4 Nutrition

Both mother and baby benefit from early breastfeeding. To the mother, suckling stimulates the release of endogenous oxytocin and uterine contraction thereby reducing the third stage of labour duration and regulating the neonates' temperature, leaving the resuscitaire for use by preterm and critically ill neonates. Additionally, it helps to reduce postpartum hemorrhage and increases uterine involution. This also helps the development of mammary glands for milk secretion, helps breast emptying and prevents inflammation of the breast (Mastitis) [50, 51].

Correspondingly, initiating breastfeeding early can save millions of neonates, their gut gets colonized with good microbiota, which promotes the immune development of the child. It also promotes growth and prevents stunting. Therefore, the midwife must ensure the mother initiates breastfeeding within the first hour of birth [52, 53].

Equally important is the care of the cord. Being a key area for introducing infection to the child, asepsis must be maintained around the cord. Regulatory bodies recommend dry cord care until its detachment which is faster compared to the use of antibiotic gels. However, chlorhexidine gel is recommended for prevention in situations where strict sterility cannot be maintained, thus chlorhexidine provides the advantage of antibiotic cover. Handwashing is the single most effective means to prevent the spread of infection to both the mother and the child. The midwife must instruct the mother and all managing the baby on the importance of hand hygiene. Endeavor to wash hands before and after taking care of the infant, after a diaper change [54].

3.2 A guided approach to assessing the newborn

Midwives perform a newborn examination at birth detect abnormality early and institute treatment quickly. Mothers are gratified to know how well their baby is doing and might need to learn how to examine their babies It is thus expedient that the midwife conducts the following examination of the baby beginning from head to toe.

The head: most babies are born headfirst and so the head is subject to injury as it navigates the birth canal. The risk of caput succedaneum and cephalhematoma with bruises and sometimes scalpel injuries from cesarean section. Show the position of the sutures. And the time they close. The posterior fontanels close at 18 months. and the posterior fontanel fuses at six weeks. When the anterior fontanel is sunken Adequate feeding will prevent dehydration.

The eyes: check the appearance of the eyes and their movement. Teach mothers to look at the baby's eyes while feeding. The newborn begins to follow objects at six meters and can see up to 12 meters.

The mouth: for tongue tie and false tooth which can fall off while feeding to prevent asphyxiation of the infant. The presence of cleft lip and palate and micrognathia [55]. For many mothers, it is a frightening experience. Therefore, they require the support of the midwife, family, and significant others. Following the examination, breastfeeding must begin within the first hour of birth. It provides nourishment and bonding between mother and baby [56].

Midwives concentrate on meeting the physiologic as well as the emotional and psychological needs of mothers, especially mothers of preterm and extreme preterm neonates. The distress of physical and emotional separation of mothers from their babies is traumatizing, contributing to emotional instability and depression [57].

Attention must be given to mothers of sick neonates to avoid losing them. Supported and informed mothers contribute better to the care of their newborns, and their well-being encourages lactation and the treatment of the neonate.

Note that the midwife conducts a complete physical examination of the child, and notifies the mother and results are recorded in the delivery notes [58].

3.2.1 The second hour postpartum

Reassess the woman and baby for bonding, any discomfort or bleeding. A heavily soaked pad is a sign of postpartum hemorrhage. The genital area should be reassessed under good lighting and if necessary, an ultrasound scan done to rule out any retained product. The perineal pad should be observed every 15 minutes until the lochia is normal. The midwife must ensure the bladder is empty with active management of the third stage of labour.

3.2.2 Observe breastfeeding and provide appropriate support

Adopting a proper breastfeeding position will encourage correct latching and the baby will get adequate nourishment and not suckle air. This will also reduce soreness or cracked nipples.

3.2.3 Nutrition

The mother should be given a warm nourishing meal with enough fluid. This will help replenish energy. Many mothers may eat little due to a mixture of emotions and fatigue. However, they should be encouraged to take liberal oral fluids to support lactation [59].

3.2.4 Sleep and rest

Most women sleep off immediately after delivery. They should be made comfortable in the lying-in wards to support rest from the strain of labour especially women with difficulty sleeping in the past. Early rest is necessary for the new mother to settle quickly into her new role of nourishing the infant. It may be difficult to restrain visitors [60].

3.2.5 Immunization

Colostrum is the first immunization the baby receives, therefore establishing breastfeeding early will ensure that. The midwife must ensure to give immunization according to local policy. The mother is educated on the importance of early childhood immunization and where and how to access same. Immunization against tuberculosis and hepatitis B is recommended within the first 24 hours. However, where that is not possible, the child should be immunized as soon as possible afterwards [61, 62].

3.2.6 Contraception

Contraceptives are a sure protection against unplanned and unintended pregnancies. And the postpartum period is the best time to make the most of its gains. Exclusive breastfeeding in the absence of menstruation amenorrhoea can guarantee protection from pregnancy.

Nevertheless, most contraceptives are safe and highly effective for use in the immediate postpartum period, the midwife can thus introduce mothers to them. Postpartum intrauterine contraception (PPIUC) can be inserted immediately to provide long-term protection. The woman enjoys the added benefit of immediate service, cost-saving from not having to return for the service. Where this is not readily available, the woman must be encouraged to return for family planning [63].

Commencing contraceptives in the immediate postpartum period is easier due to the ease and proximity to family planning services at the place of delivery. The woman ovulates 2 weeks before the next menstruation and because menses have not resumed, many women become pregnant within this period and are at risk of unintended, unplanned pregnancy and associated abortion risk. Therefore, encouraging early postpartum contraceptive uptake [64].

3.3 Subsequent care

Global health authorities recommend up to four postnatal visits: within 24 hours of birth, 3–7 days, 2 weeks, and 6 weeks postpartum. At each, both child and mother should be thoroughly examined, educated, and counseled on measures to cope with the phase of growth. Both the child and mother are examined, and results are recorded. Counseling on nutrition, exclusive breastfeeding, urination, lochia, and the uterus is assessed noting uterine height, involution, perineal and hand hygiene and how they are coping with childcare. The neonate is equally assessed for any deviation from normal. He is weighed and details are documented on the growth chart [45, 65].

4. Challenges to providing effective postpartum midwifery care

The postnatal period is challenging for clients and caregivers. Midwives as carers share in the emotions of their clients and experience the emotions of their clients and because they are empathetic to their plight, they suffer anxiety and psychological stress. This has the propensity to interfere with the quality of care they render. Midwives must adapt quickly, be resilient, communicate and foster support for the mothers. The inability to separate self from the problem would lead to a crisis or worsen the existing crisis. Communication is a key factor to support midwives experiencing the stress of caring for postpartum mothers. Effective communication with peers and support systems can reduce tension of this kind [66].

Midwives at the lead are associated with improved postnatal maternal outcomes, they protect and preserve the integrity of mothers, but experience decreased adverse events [67]. However, midwives still face challenges while rendering this care. Midwives encounter while giving postnatal the issues of continuity, collaboration, and communication quality. Though there are concerns relating to individual perceptions of midwives regards implementing midwifery-led actions, the accrued benefits to postpartum women and the ease of adapting such models are undeniable [68].

There are also challenges to providing care consistently in this model related to time constraints, the unpredictability of labour and the inconsistency of mothers. Other challenges include inadequate workforce and empowerment of midwives and lack of support from facility management [68].

Implementing quality midwifery care is preceded by adequate planning and implementation of care standards. Therefore, midwives must be conversant with unit and facility protocol and work at sustaining the same. Training midwives in that light will sustain the process and reduce distress [69].

5. Strategies to combat postnatal challenges

Recognizing that postpartum women sometimes abruptly get into this stage without adequate preparation, they require huge support mostly from their caregivers to overcome these challenges. And because women present with differing needs, a one-size-fits-all approach will not solve the problem. Adopting the individualized care approach will suffice [70]. This brief section will discuss client-related strategies and health worker-related strategies geared toward supporting the smooth transition and function of postpartum women.

While focusing on the client-related strategy, it is critical to improve the education of women/families by re-enforcing educational content through the provision of information leaflets with opportunities to clarify misconceptions and questions. This will increase women's self-confidence, self-efficacy, and satisfaction [71]. Other educational care involves the need for compliance with medication, appointments, and follow-up care. Supportive care will enhance breastfeeding and the care of the baby [72].

On the other hand, changing times require improvement in care outcomes and input from workers. Midwives communicate skill, competence and professionalism while being sensitive to client's needs and prioritize patient care rather than organizational priorities [73]. There appears increased progressive knowledge of the client due to the ease of assessing information and technological improvements. Caregivers must respond adequately and professionally to the information needs of clients, bridging the knowledge gap with effective learning and dissemination of life-preserving and lifesaving information [74].

Appropriate weight gain in pregnancy is beneficial to the health of the mother and fetus. Though prenatal and postpartum weight gain or loss appears associated with the sociodemographic characteristics of many women [75], lack of weight control is associated with obesity, and gestational diabetes that could complicate fetal and maternal pregnancy outcomes. Which could lead to stress, inadequate coping the development of Type II diabetes mellitus and poor health outcomes [76].

To prevent this, women are therefore advised to adhere to adequate nutrition during and after pregnancy. The combination of diet and exercise is a good strategy for maintaining ideal weight and health during postpartum [77]. Moreover, the maintenance of ideal weight contributes to self-esteem and confidence building. It portends better well-being and welfare for the mother and baby [1].

Paying special attention to caring for women with special needs or medical conditions, and building trusts is yet another strategy. Women with or without a history of pregnancy-induced hypertension can develop postpartum pre-eclampsia. A higher risk associated with pregnancy-induced hypertension occurs within 48 hours postpartum. Therefore, such women must receive closer blood pressure monitoring with laboratory investigations. They also will benefit from shorter and more frequent checks within seven days of delivery [78].

Strategy to cope with pain involves judicious and appropriate use of analgesics and increased rest periods, especially for women who had a cesarean section or instrumental deliveries [68, 79]. Exercise also promotes mental health as well as physiologic return and function [80]. Every visit allows a review of their emotional and psychological state will drive client-centred care. An attentive listener can decipher more information from the pieces of information obtained during conversations [65].

Improve the midwives' attitude to clients. Many clients have developed negative impressions of the manner health workers deal with them. This goes a long way to determine their acceptance and adherence to treatment instructions. Safe delivery of their babies thus paves the way to escape from the facility and health workers. Midwives must develop a good work ethic and attitude toward patients. And desist from breaking the care continuum through negative attitudes [81].

Improved capacity for patient and patient information management is key to overcoming postpartum care challenges. So is the need for organizational buy-in institutionalizing patient care standards, policies, and protocols [32]. Health organizations and regulatory bodies must provide leadership and direction to achieve a safer healthcare system, and service. Ensure a conducive work environment with tools where providers can give competent and quality care that promotes maternal well-being and health that benefits the family and society. This is achievable with adequate budgetary provision and health financing [82].

6. Conclusion

Challenges that postpartum encounters can limit the full enjoyment of the childbearing experience. Psychologic concerns can be difficult to identify and manage. All mothers should be offered skilled maternity care regardless of economic, social, and environmental status. Postnatal mothers should be offered contraceptive counsel and service at each visit and given support. Make an informed contraceptive choice. Then women who have adopted a method are reviewed and asked how they are faring with their choice. Mothers will benefit from cervical cancer counseling and screening tests using the midwifery model of care.

Acknowledgements

I wish to acknowledge the special support and contributions of my husband Mr. Paul Ochala and to UNICAF University Zambia.

Conflict of interest

The author declares no conflict of interest.

Author details

Ejura Ochala
Federal Medical Center, UNICAF University, Abuja, Nigeria

*Address all correspondence to: ejujennifer@yahoo.com

IntechOpen

© 2023 The Author(s). Licensee IntechOpen. This chapter is distributed under the terms of the Creative Commons Attribution License (http://creativecommons.org/licenses/by/3.0), which permits unrestricted use, distribution, and reproduction in any medium, provided the original work is properly cited.

References

[1] Finlayson K, Crossland N, Bonet M, Downe S. What matters to women in the postnatal period: A meta-synthesis of qualitative studies. PLoS One. 2020;**15**(4):e0231415

[2] Kikuchi K, Yasuoka J, Nanishi K, Ahmed A, Nohara Y, Nishikitani M, et al. Postnatal care could be the key to improving the continuum of care in maternal and child health in Ratanakiri, Cambodia. PLoS One. 2018;**13**(6):e0198829

[3] Spelke B, Erika Werner MD. The fourth trimester of pregnancy: Committing to maternal health and well-being postpartum. Rhode Island Medical Journal. 2018;**101**(8):30-33

[4] Kazma JM, van den Anker J, Allegaert K, Dallmann A, Ahmadzia HK. Anatomical and physiological alterations of pregnancy. Journal of Pharmacokinetics and Pharmacodynamics. 2020;**47**(4):271-285

[5] Martin C, Rokibullah R, Sofinia H. The physiological changes in the postpartum period after childbirth. Asian Journal of Social and Humanities. 2022;**1**(03):105-118

[6] Critchley CJ. Physical therapy is an important component of postpartum care in the fourth trimester. Physical Therapy. 2022;**102**(5):pzac021

[7] Bjelica A, Cetkovic N, Trninic-Pjevic A, Mladenovic-Segedi L. The phenomenon of pregnancy—A psychological view. Ginekologia Polska. 2018;**89**(2):102-106

[8] Atkinson L, Teychenne M. Psychological, social, and behavioural changes during pregnancy: Implications for physical activity and exercise. In: Exercise and Physical Activity during Pregnancy and Postpartum. Cham: Springer; 2022. pp. 21-45

[9] García-León MÁ, Caparrós-González RA, Romero-González B, González-Perez R, Peralta-Ramírez I. Resilience as a protective factor in pregnancy and puerperium: Its relationship with the psychological state, and with hair cortisol concentrations. Midwifery. 2019;**75**:138-145

[10] Marques R, Monteiro F, Canavarro MC, Fonseca A. The role of emotion regulation difficulties in the relationship between attachment representations and depressive and anxiety symptoms in the postpartum period. Journal of Affective Disorders. 2018;**238**:39-46

[11] Cole JC, Olkkola M, Zarrin HE, Berger K, Moldenhauer JS. Universal postpartum mental health screening for parents of newborns with prenatally diagnosed birth defects. Journal of Obstetric, Gynecologic & Neonatal Nursing. 2018;**47**(1):84-93

[12] Qamar N, Ali MA, Bashir K, Asif R, Naveed N, Zafar K. Prevalence of postpartum depression and its risk factors among Pakistani females. MedERA-Journal of CMH LMC and IOD. 2022;**4**(2):78-82

[13] Ohara M, Okada T, Aleksic B, Morikawa M, Kubota C, Nakamura Y, et al. Social support helps protect against perinatal bonding failure and depression among mothers: A prospective cohort study. Scientific Reports. 2017;**7**(1):1-8

[14] Obrochta CA, Chambers C, Bandoli G. Psychological distress in

pregnancy and postpartum. Women and Birth. 2020;**33**(6):583-591

[15] Bauer AE, Maegbaek ML, Liu X, Wray NR, Sullivan PF, Miller WC, et al. Familiality of psychiatric disorders and risk of postpartum psychiatric episodes: A population-based cohort study. American Journal of Psychiatry. 2018;**175**(8):783-791

[16] Law KH, Jackson B, Guelfi K, Nguyen T, Dimmock JA. Understanding and alleviating maternal postpartum distress: Perspectives from first-time mothers in Australia. Social Science & Medicine. 2018;**204**:59-66

[17] Chrzan-Dętkoś M, Walczak-Kozłowska T, Pietkiewicz A, Żołnowska J. Improvement of the breastfeeding self-efficacy and postpartum mental health after lactation consultations–observational study. Midwifery. 2021;**94**:102905

[18] Arefadib N, Cooklin A, Nicholson J, Shafiei T. Postnatal depression and anxiety screening and management by maternal and child health nurses in community settings: A scoping review. Midwifery. 2021;**100**:103039

[19] Gilden J, Molenaar NM, Smit AK, Hoogendijk WJ, Rommel AS, Kamperman AM, et al. Mother-to-infant bonding in women with postpartum psychosis and severe postpartum depression: A clinical cohort study. Journal of Clinical Medicine. 2020;**9**(7):2291

[20] Lutkiewicz K, Bieleninik Ł, Cieślak M, Bidzan M. Maternal–infant bonding and its relationships with maternal depressive symptoms, stress, and anxiety in the early postpartum period in a polish sample. International Journal of Environmental Research and Public Health. 2020;**17**(15):5427

[21] Byrne V, Egan J, Mac Neela P, Sarma K. What about me? The loss of self through the experience of traumatic childbirth. Midwifery. 2017;**51**:1-11

[22] de Vries NE, Stramrood CA, Sligter LM, Sluijs AM, van Pampus MG. Midwives' practices and knowledge about fear of childbirth and postpartum posttraumatic stress disorder. Women and Birth. 2020;**33**(1):e95-e104

[23] Browne PD, Bossenbroek R, Kluft A, Van Tetering EM, De Weerth C. Prenatal anxiety and depression: Treatment uptake, barriers, and facilitators in midwifery care. Journal of Women's Health. 2021;**30**(8):1116-1126

[24] Pope J, Redsell S, Houghton C, Matvienko-Sikar K. Healthcare professionals' experiences and perceptions of providing support for mental health during the period from pregnancy to two years postpartum. Midwifery. 2023;**118**:103581

[25] Grylka-Baeschlin S, Iglesias C, Erdin R, Pehlke-Milde J. Evaluation of a midwifery network to guarantee outpatient postpartum care: A mixed methods study. BMC Health Services Research. 2020;**20**:1-12

[26] McGuinness C, Mottl-Santiago J, Nass M, Siegel L, Onyekwu OC, Cruikshank A, et al. Dyadic care mobile units: A collaborative midwifery and pediatric response to the COVID-19 pandemic. Journal of Midwifery & Women's Health. 2022;**67**(6):714-719

[27] Frederiksen MS, Schmied V, Overgaard C. Supportive encounters during pregnancy and the postnatal period: An ethnographic study of care experiences of parents in a vulnerable position. Journal of Clinical Nursing. 2021;**30**(15-16):2386-2398

[28] Domínguez-Solís E, Lima-Serrano M, Lima-Rodriguez JS. Non-pharmacological interventions to reduce anxiety in pregnancy, labour and postpartum: A systematic review. Midwifery. 2021;**102**:103126

[29] Sangsawang B, Deoisres W, Hengudomsub P, Sangsawang N. Effectiveness of psychosocial support provided by midwives and family on preventing postpartum depression among first-time adolescent mothers at 3-month follow-up: A randomised controlled trial. Journal of Clinical Nursing. 2022;**31**(5-6):689-702

[30] He Y, He H, Tang C. Effect of psychological nursing intervention on abnormal-induced labor of fetus during puerperium: Study on the effects of anxiety, depression, and life events. Computational and Mathematical Methods in Medicine. 2022;**2022**

[31] Al-abri K, Armitage CJ, Edge D. Views of healthcare professionals and service users regarding anti-, peri-and post-natal depression in Oman. Journal of Psychiatric and Mental Health Nursing. 2023;**30**(4):795-812

[32] Roets L, Chelagat D, Joubert A. Strategies to improve postnatal care in Kenya: A qualitative study. International Journal of Africa Nursing Sciences. 2018;**9**:62-67

[33] Perzow SE, Hennessey EMP, Hoffman MC, Grote NK, Davis EP, Hankin BL. Mental health of pregnant and postpartum women in response to the COVID-19 pandemic. Journal of Affective Disorders Reports. 2021;**4**:100123

[34] International Confederation of Midwives. Philosophy and model of midwifery care. Strengthening Midwifery Globally. 2014;**1**(1):1-3

[35] Mortensen B, Lieng M, Diep LM, Lukasse M, Atieh K, Fosse E. Improving maternal and neonatal health by a midwife-led continuity model of care–an observational study in one governmental hospital in Palestine. EClinicalMedicine. 2019;**10**:84-91

[36] Okereke E, Ishaku SM, Unumeri G, Mohammed B, Ahonsi B. Reducing maternal and newborn mortality in Nigeria—A qualitative study of stakeholders' perceptions about the performance of community health workers and the introduction of community midwifery at primary healthcare level. Human Resources for Health. 2019;**17**(1):1-9

[37] Tikkanen R, Gunja MZ, FitzGerald M, Zephyrin L. Maternal mortality and maternity care in the United States compared to 10 other developed countries. The Commonwealth Fund. 2020;**10**:1-17

[38] Mose A, Fikadu Y, Zewdie A, Haile K, Shitu S, Wasie Kasahun A, et al. Pregnant women's perception of midwifery-led continuity care model in Ethiopia: A qualitative study. BMC Women's Health. 2023;**23**(1):1-8

[39] Choudhary S, Jelly P, Mahala P. Models of maternity care: Continuity of midwifery care. International Journal of Reproduction, Contraception, Obstetrics and Gynecology. 2020;**9**(6):2667

[40] Iliadou M, Papadakaki M, Sioti E, Giaxi P, Leontitsi E, Petelos E, et al. Addressing mental health issues among migrant and refugee pregnant women: A call for action. European Journal of Midwifery. 2019;**3**:1-8

[41] Baghini FK, Iranifard E, Roudsari RL, Najmabadi KM. The role of midwives in Women's empowerment: A narrative review. Journal of

Midwifery & Reproductive Health. 2023;**11**(3):3767-3781

[42] Botfield JR, Tulloch M, Contziu H, Phipps H, Bateson D, Wright SM, et al. Contraception provision in the postpartum period: Knowledge, views, and practices of midwives. Women and Birth. 2021;**34**(1):e1-e6

[43] Woodley SJ, Hay-Smith EJC. Narrative review of pelvic floor muscle training for childbearing women—Why, when, what, and how. International Urogynecology Journal. 2021;**32**(7):1977-1988

[44] Finnbogadóttir H, Torkelsson E, Christensen CB, Persson EK. Midwife's experiences of meeting pregnant women who are exposed to Intimate-Partner Violence at in-hospital prenatal ward: A qualitative study. European Journal of Midwifery. 2020;**4**

[45] World Health Organization and Jhpiego. Postnatal Care for Mothers and Newborns Highlights from the World Health Organization 2013 Guidelines, WHO/RHR/15.05. 2015

[46] Othman ALH, Sayyed TM, Gomaa AM, Elnasr IA. A normal pattern of uterine involution using symphysis-fundal distance. Menoufia Medical Journal. 2022;**35**(1):270

[47] Widström AM, Brimdyr K, Svensson K, Cadwell K, Nissen E. Skin-to-skin contact the first hour after birth, underlying implications, and clinical practice. Acta Paediatrica. 2019;**108**(7):1192-1204

[48] Costa S, Menzella N, Vento G, Barnea ER, FIGO Childbirth and Postpartum Hemorrhage Committee, Beyeza J, et al. FIGO good practice recommendations: Bundle of care to reduce neonatal mortality and improve outcomes after preterm and term delivery. International Journal of Gynecology & Obstetrics. 2023;**163**:68-73

[49] Salam MW, Hye MA, Kundu JK, Ahmed S. Successful 'kangaroo mother care': A necessity for preterm low birth weight babies in rural hospital settings in Bangladesh. Bangladesh Journal of Medical Science. 2022;**21**(4):875

[50] Al Sabati SY, Mousa O. Effect of early initiation of breastfeeding on the uterine consistency and the amount of vaginal blood loss during early postpartum period. Nursing Primary Care. 2019;**3**(3):2-7

[51] Safari K, Saeed AA, Hasan SS, Moghaddam-Banaem L. The effect of mother and newborn early skin-to-skin contact on initiation of breastfeeding, newborn temperature, and duration of third stage of labour. International Breastfeeding Journal. 2018;**13**(1):1-8

[52] Lyons KE, Ryan CA, Dempsey EM, Ross RP, Stanton C. Breast milk, a source of beneficial microbes and associated benefits for infant health. Nutrients. 2020;**12**(4):1039-1069

[53] Muldiasman M, Kusharisupeni K, Laksminingsih E, Besral B. Can early initiation to breastfeeding prevent stunting in 6-59 months old children? Journal of Health Research. 2018

[54] Abbaszadeh F, Hajizadeh Z, Seraji P, Sadat Z. Comparing the impacts of topical chlorhexidine and dry cord care on umbilical cord separation time among neonates. Nursing and Midwifery Studies. 2018;**7**(2):62

[55] Rutter C. Examination of the newborn baby at birth. The Midwife's Labour and Birth Handbook. 2017:105-121. DOI: 10.1002/9781119235064.ch5

[56] Saco MC, Coca KP, Marcacine KO, Abuchaim ÉDSV, Abrão ACFDV. Skin-to-skin contact followed by breastfeeding in the first hour of life: Associated factors and influences on exclusive breastfeeding. Texto & Contexto-Enfermagem. 2019;**28**:86-99

[57] Fowler C, Green J, Elliott D, Petty J, Whiting L. The forgotten mothers of extremely preterm babies: A qualitative study. Journal of Clinical Nursing. 2019;**28**(11-12):2124-2134

[58] Nakphong MK, Sacks E, Opot J, Sudhinaraset M. Separating newborns from mothers and maternal consent for newborn care and the association with health care satisfaction, use and breastfeeding: Findings from a longitudinal survey in Kenya. medRxiv. 2020 2020-10

[59] Aparicio E, Jardí C, Bedmar C, Pallejà M, Basora J, Arija V, et al. Nutrient intake during pregnancy and post-partum: ECLIPSES study. Nutrients. 2020;**12**(5):1325

[60] Kalmbach DA, O'Brien LM, Pitts DAS, Sagong C, Arnett LK, Harb NC, et al. Mother-to-infant bonding is associated with maternal insomnia, snoring, cognitive arousal, and infant sleep problems and colic. Behavioral Sleep Medicine. 2022;**20**(4):393-409

[61] Camacho-Morales A, Caba M, García-Juárez M, Caba-Flores MD, Viveros-Contreras R, Martínez-Valenzuela C. Breastfeeding contributes to physiological immune programming in the newborn. Frontiers in Pediatrics. 2021;**9**:744104

[62] Chirumbolo S, Vella A, Peroni DG. The extra-lymphoid compartment of breast milk: Not a simple transfer of passive immunization. Journal of Leucocyte Biology. 2021;**109**(4):693-695

[63] Cooper M, Cameron S. Postpartum contraception. ScienceDirect' Obstetrics, Gynaecology & Reproductive Medicine. 2018;**28**(6):183-185

[64] Sey-Sawo J, Adeyemo FO, Okojie OH. Effects of postpartum family planning counselling on contraceptives knowledge, attitude and intention among women attending a general hospital in the Gambia: A randomized controlled trial. Open Access Journal of Contraception. 2023;**4**:61-72

[65] World Health Organization. WHO Recommendations on Antenatal Care for a Positive Pregnancy Experience. World Health Organization; 2016

[66] Bradfield Z, Hauck Y, Homer CS, Sweet L, Wilson AN, Szabo RA, et al. Midwives' experiences of providing maternity care during the COVID-19 pandemic in Australia. Women and Birth. 2022;**35**(3):262-271

[67] Gidaszewski B, Khajehei M, Gibbs E, Chua SC. Comparison of the effect of caseload midwifery program and standard midwifery-led care on primiparous birth outcomes: A retrospective cohort matching study. Midwifery. 2019;**69**:10-16

[68] Dharni N, Essex H, Bryant MJ, Cronin de Chavez A, Willan K, Farrar D, et al. The key components of a successful model of midwifery-led continuity of carer, without continuity at birth: Findings from a qualitative implementation evaluation. BMC Pregnancy and Childbirth. 2021;**21**:1-11

[69] Styles C, Kearney L, George K. Implementation and upscaling of midwifery continuity of care: The experience of midwives and obstetricians. Women and Birth. 2020;**33**(4):343-351

[70] Peahl AF, Novara A, Heisler M, Dalton VK, Moniz MH, Smith RD. Patient preferences for prenatal and postpartum care delivery: A survey of postpartum women. Obstetrics and Gynecology. 2020;**135**(5):1038

[71] Jiao N, Zhu L, Chong YS, Chan WCS, Luo N, Wang W, et al. Web-based versus home-based postnatal psychoeducational interventions for first-time mothers: A randomised controlled trial. International Journal of Nursing Studies. 2019;**99**:103385-103396

[72] Church L. Quiet time during postpartum hospitalization can improve rest, bonding, and breastfeeding. Nursing for Women's Health. 2020. DOI: 10.1016/j.nwh.2020.03.002

[73] Sacks E, Finlayson K, Brizuela V, Crossland N, Ziegler D, Sauvé C, et al. Factors that influence uptake of routine postnatal care: Findings on women's perspectives from a qualitative evidence synthesis. PLoS One. 2022;**17**(8):1-30. e0270264

[74] Chiba Y, Hayashi R, Kita Y, Takeshita M. Care provided by midwives and the unmet needs of pregnant and postpartum women: A qualitative study of Japanese mothers. Heliyon. 2023

[75] Djaković I, Soljačić-Vraneš H, Kuna K. Weight gain in pregnancy and weight retention after birth. Open Access Macedonian Journal of Medical Sciences. 2019;7(4):614

[76] Dolatian M, Sharifi N, Mahmoodi Z, Fathnezhad-Kazemi A, Bahrami-Vazir E, Rashidian T. Weight gain during pregnancy and its associated factors: A path analysis. Nursing Open. 2020;7(5):1568-1577

[77] Adegboye ARA, Linne YM. Diet or exercise, or both, for weight reduction in women after childbirth. Cochrane Database of Systematic Reviews. 2013;(7)

[78] Paladine HL, Blenning CE, Strangas Y. Postpartum care: An approach to the fourth trimester. American Family Physician. 2019;**100**(8):485-491

[79] Schmied V, Cooke M, Gutwein R, Steinlein E, Homer C. An evaluation of strategies to improve the quality and content of hospital-based postnatal care in a metropolitan Australian hospital. Journal of Clinical Nursing. 2009;**18**(13):1850-1861

[80] Li Q. The effects of yoga exercise on pelvic floor rehabilitation of postpartum women. Journal of Healthcare Engineering. 2022;**2022**

[81] Ochieng CA, Odhiambo AS. Barriers to formal health care seeking during pregnancy, childbirth, and postnatal period: A qualitative study in Siaya County in rural Kenya. BMC Pregnancy and Childbirth. 2019;**19**:339

[82] Dahlen HG, Drandic D, Shah N, Cadee F. Supporting midwifery is the answer to the wicked problems in maternity care. The Lancet Global Health. 2022;**10**(7):e951-e952

Chapter 6

Perspective Chapter: Challenges to Postnatal Care in Sub-Saharan Africa – A Review

Juliana Yartey Enos, Richard Dickson Amoako, Samuel Kweku Enos, Beatrice Hayford and Edem Magdalene Tette

Abstract

The postnatal period remains the most at-risk period for the mother-infant dyad. Most maternal and neonatal deaths occur in the immediate postnatal period, contributing to the greatest burden of child mortality. Appropriate care for mothers and newborns during this critical period is essential to improve their survival. However, access to quality care during this period remains a challenge, especially in resource-limited settings. This chapter examines challenges to postnatal care (PNC) in sub-Saharan Africa (SSA), drawing on existing evidence. A comprehensive review of critically appraised literature was undertaken. The findings indicate suboptimal uptake of PNC, resulting in high maternal and neonatal morbidity and mortality in the postnatal period. Challenges to the delivery of quality PNC include poor healthcare infrastructure and access to basic health services, and underlying structural determinants such as widespread poverty, illiteracy, harmful cultural practices, marginalization of women, and inadequate political will by governments. These challenges underscore the need for intensified efforts to improve PNC in the region. Innovative approaches to increasing demand and reaching mothers with PNC services within communities are critically needed to improve access and utilization of PNC in SSA, improve maternal and child health outcomes, and contribute to achieving the sustainable development goals in 2030.

Keywords: postnatal care, maternal and newborn care, neonatal care, health systems, sub-Saharan Africa

1. Introduction

The postnatal period, which starts after birth and lasts for 42 days, is a crucial phase for the health and survival of the mother and the baby [1]. Most newborn fatalities occur within the first month of life, with three-quarters of these deaths occurring within the first 24 hours [2]. In addition, two-thirds of maternal deaths in low- and middle-income countries also occur in the postnatal period [3]. Postnatal care provides opportunities to obtain health interventions and support that are essential for the health and survival of the

IntechOpen

mother and child. These include interventions such as exclusive breastfeeding, adequate nutrition during nursing, newborn care guidance, and family planning procedures [1].

Sub-Saharan Africa (SSA) has disproportionately high rates of maternal mortality, mostly as a result of inadequate utilization of maternal healthcare throughout pregnancy, childbirth and the postnatal period [4]. Studies have demonstrated the effectiveness of maternal health services including antenatal, childbirth, and postnatal care in preventing maternal and newborn morbidity and mortality. Maternal health services provide important health information for optimal pregnancy outcomes and prompt management of health problems to reduce maternal and newborn morbidity and mortality [1, 4]. Therefore, one of the important measures for eliminating preventable causes of maternal and newborn deaths is increasing coverage of the completion of the maternal and newborn continuum of care, which includes postnatal care [5].

This chapter aims to examine the status of postnatal care in sub-Saharan Africa and the challenges associated with access and utilization by mothers. It also aims to highlight key issues, which might enable governments and stakeholders to develop effective policies and strategies to address these challenges and improve the quality and uptake of postnatal care services towards improved survival and health outcomes. Furthermore, the discussions in this chapter are critical to expanding our understanding of postnatal care in sub-Saharan Africa.

2. Status of maternal and newborn health and survival in sub-Saharan Africa

According to the global sustainable development goals (SDG) targets, by 2030, the maternal mortality ratio should be reduced to less than 70 maternal deaths per 100,000 live births, with no country having more than twice the global rate of 140 maternal deaths per 100,000 live births, and there should be no more than 12 neonatal deaths per 1000 live births, globally [5, 6]. Although progress has been made in reducing mortality rates among mothers and babies, recent evidence suggest stalled progress on preventable maternal deaths, globally [7]. For example, in 2016 alone, 7000 newborn babies died every day. Newborn deaths made up 46 per cent of all child deaths, an increase from 41 per cent in 2000 (**Figure 1**) [8].

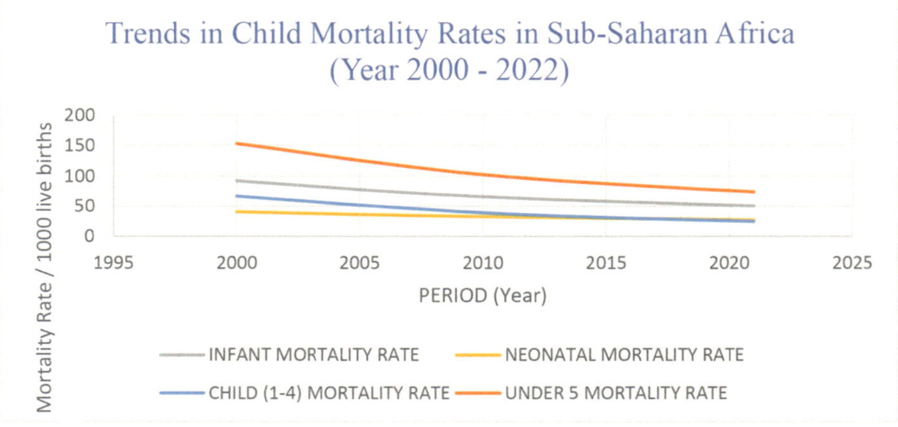

Figure 1.
Based on estimates by the United Nations inter-agency Group for Child Mortality Report, 2020 [8].

Compared to other regions, countries in the SSA region have made the least progress in lowering maternal and neonatal death rates [7, 9]. The sub-region still has the highest maternal death rate, estimated at about 542 per 100,000 live births in 2017 [10]. Since 2000, maternal death rates have decreased by 33% in a number of Sub-Saharan African countries, but the region still accounted for 70% of global maternal mortality in 2020 [11]. Also, despite making up 16% of the global population, 38% of newborn mortality takes place in Africa [8]. Between the period from 1990 to 2017, SSA recorded a 40% reduction in neonatal mortality rates, which was lower than that observed in high-income nations (55%) [12]. Despite progress, the SSA region still has a long way to go to achieve its 2030 target of zero preventable maternal, stillbirth, and neonatal deaths [5]. To achieve the 2030 targets, the region's average yearly reduction rate would have to be doubled [13]. It is important to critically appraise and understand these trends and institute appropriate measures towards achievement of the SDG targets for 2030.

3. The role of postnatal care in averting maternal and newborn deaths

Postnatal care (PNC) plays a critical role in preventing morbidity and mortality in mothers and babies [1]. In sub-Saharan Africa, the predominant causes of maternal mortality are postpartum hemorrhage, hypertensive disorders and postpartum sepsis, while infections, low birth weight and asphyxia are the main causes of newborn deaths. These infections include those that are common in preterm babies such as sepsis, meningitis, pneumonia and diarrhea, nearly all of which can be prevented or managed with appropriate PNC [1]. If care is provided as soon as the baby is born, most of the neonatal deaths that happen within the first 48 hours of life can be avoided [14, 15]. For instance, interventions such as ensuring a clean and safe delivery, which includes having clean hands, perineum, delivery surface, cord-cutting surface and instruments, proper umbilical cord care in order to minimize infections in mothers and babies, and starting breastfeeding immediately after birth might reduce maternal and neonatal infections and associated mortality significantly [14–16]. In addition, the WHO PNC recommendations promote immediate and exclusive breastfeeding, examining the mother and baby for danger signs and referring patients appropriately [14]. Early PNC interventions for neonates include kangaroo care, breastfeeding assistance, hypothermia prevention and treatment, as well as case management and referral for pneumonia [1]. For preterm infants, low birth weight babies, infants with HIV-infected mothers, and other high-risk situations such as babies with neonatal jaundice or who have recovered from birth asphyxia, acute surgical problems, genital tract abnormalities, as well as orphaned and abandoned babies, specialized PNC monitoring is also recommended [1]. By providing key assistance that identifies warning signals, promotes beneficial behaviors, and streamlines referral procedures, postnatal care (PNC) plays a critical role in lowering morbidity and mortality rates in mothers and babies [1]. Given that interventions during the postnatal period can prevent a significant proportion of maternal and neonatal deaths, increasing efforts to improve uptake of postnatal care is particularly crucial for lowering maternal and neonatal mortality rates [4, 5].

4. Maternal healthcare utilization in sub-Saharan Africa

Since 2015, there have been considerable improvements in maternal healthcare utilization in sub-Saharan African countries [17]. Yet challenges remain in ensuring universal access and utilization of maternal health services. Differences in care-seeking habits and poor usage of maternal and newborn health services are blamed for sub-Saharan Africa's slower progress in improving maternal, neonatal and child health outcomes [18]. For instance, just 48% of women in the region deliver their babies with the help of skilled attendants, compared to 72% of women globally [19]. Additionally, SSA nations continue to see persistent disparities in access to, and utilization of high-quality services, with notable access gaps between the poor and non-poor populations [20, 21]. Socioeconomic status and the location of the mother's residence have a major impact on the use of maternal, neonatal and child healthcare, with persistent wealth-related disparities [9]. The least equitable interventions, according to a study of 54 low- and middle-income countries, were four or more ANC visits and skilled birth attendance coverage. The lowest quintile (32%), in comparison to the richest quintile (84%), had lower mean skilled-birth attendance coverage [22]. This situation has a significant impact on postnatal care utilization.

5. Determinants of maternal and newborn healthcare utilization in sub-Saharan Africa

Several studies have documented various facilitators and barriers to women's access to healthcare during pregnancy, childbirth and the postnatal period in SSA [23]. These determinants occur at the individual, health system and contextual levels.

5.1 Individual factors

At the individual level, maternal age, educational attainment, occupation, income, religion, family structure, information accessibility, location of residence, health awareness, and decision-making authority are all factors that affect maternal and newborn healthcare access and utilization [24]. For instance, exposure to local media and information sources has a positive impact on maternal and neonatal care utilization [25], and frequent broadcast of the benefits of birthing at a healthcare facility encourage mothers to adopt health facility deliveries [25].

5.2 Health system factors

At the health system level, maternal healthcare utilization in sub-Saharan Africa is influenced by factors that include accessibility to healthcare facilities, perceived quality of care, financial cost, timeliness of care, availability of drugs and equipment, and emergency care [26, 27]. Healthcare quality considerations include human resource availability, the population-to-healthcare-professionals ratio, and service accessibility [28, 29]. Women are more likely to use maternal healthcare services if they reside in areas with high-performing and high-quality health systems. However, some studies have also reported either a negative association between distance and maternal healthcare utilization or no significant association [29, 30]. In these instances, increased rates of facility delivery were attributed to contextual factors such as access to health facilities within communities, which appeared to have an impact on immediate postnatal care [29].

5.3 Contextual factors

Individual and health system-level variables reflect "upstream" contextual variables that are ingrained in larger social systems. For instance, discussions of the impact of women's autonomy and decision-making power on maternal healthcare frequently take place within the context of prevalent masculine beliefs or local cultural norms [31]. Pregnancy and childbirth have typically offered women in sub-Saharan Africa an opportunity to establish their worth and stake an assertion on social status through childbirth [32]. In cases where a woman gives birth without external support, she is held in high esteem. Such perspectives may influence the decision of childbirth at home without the support of any health professional. Also, in some communities, local beliefs prevent health facility deliveries as they are considered unacceptable [33]. Expectant mothers, out of fear, choose to appease their families by having home births in order not to endanger their lives and that of their babies [33]. These beliefs make it difficult for mothers to freely access maternal health care. In some traditional settings, the consent of the woman's spouse is often required to access care at a healthcare facility [34]. Some men insist on home birth in order to prevent their wives from being attended to by male health personnel [34]. For women who live in vulnerable environments such as in conflict and war situations, the risk of being kidnapped, raped or killed makes it impractical to travel to a health facility for childbirth and PNC services [35]. Similarly, the dysfunction of the political and governance institutions that control health systems may have a direct or indirect impact on health systems. Contextual-level factors strongly explain variability in individual access to healthcare and health outcomes [36].

6. Postnatal care utilization in sub-Saharan Africa

Data from Demographic and Health Surveys conducted in 23 African nations show that less than 13% of women in sub-Saharan Africa receive postnatal care within two days of childbirth, and only one-third of women give birth in a medical institution [37]. From 2006 to 2018, the pooled magnitude of postnatal care service utilization in sub-Saharan African countries was 52.48% with the highest utilization in the central region of Africa (73.5%) and the lowest utilization in the eastern region (31.7%) [23]. Progress is being made and in many countries, a significant proportion of women increasingly access PNC [5]. However, postnatal care utilization remains low within the continuum of care.

7. Challenges to postnatal care in sub-Sahara Africa

Several challenges to PNC in sub-Saharan Africa have been documented [23].

One of the key challenges associated with postnatal care in SSA is a lack of access to basic healthcare services [23]. Many women in the region live in remote, rural areas that lack adequate healthcare facilities [35, 38]. Healthcare facilities in the region are often understaffed, and the staff available may not be adequately trained to provide the care that is needed [18]. The facilities also lack basic medical supplies such as drugs and equipment, which can make it difficult for healthcare workers to provide the care that is needed, and for women to receive appropriate care during the postnatal period [18, 38].

Even when postnatal care services are available, a variety of sociocultural barriers prevent mothers and their newborns from accessing these services. These include household barriers related to the educational level and health literacy of mothers and other family members, the influence of sociocultural beliefs and practices, and women's autonomy and decision-making power [39]. Specific examples of sociocultural barriers to postnatal care utilization include cultural beliefs about the 40 days following childbirth, during which mothers and babies should stay indoors [40], misconceptions about the importance of postnatal care, and a lack of knowledge about postnatal care and its benefits [35].

At the individual level, a woman's education and literacy level, occupation, income and access to information influence her access and utilization of PNC. At the health system level, the cost of health services, transportation, accessibility, travel time and distance to healthcare facilities all influence utilization of PNC. The functionality and standard of health systems at the community level, the standard of care provided at the facility and concerns about the quality of care, including the attitudes of health workers, their skills, resources, workload and effect on the quality of care, and the cultural acceptability of services all influence women's decision to seek PNC [28, 35].

Socioeconomic characteristics such as place of residence, cultural attitudes, gender norms, women's autonomy and empowerment, wealth or poverty levels in the community, levels of education at the community level, population density, and the government's contribution to healthcare spending, and gross national income per capita are contextual variables that affect the utilization of postnatal care [25, 29]. The extent of poverty, socioeconomic development and infrastructure, including poor roads and transportation, can also make it difficult for women to reach healthcare facilities, even if they are available [18, 35, 38].

Utilization of postnatal care is correlated with several of these factors predictably and consistently. For instance, it is well known that women are more likely to use maternal healthcare if they reside in regions or countries with higher socioeconomic or educational standards. it is also well known that women who reside in rural regions are less likely to use postnatal care and other maternal healthcare services. Many women in the region live in poverty and do not have the resources, information, autonomy and decision-making power to access care during the postnatal period. Discrimination and other social factors also make it difficult for women to access and receive the care they need [18, 35, 38].

Contextual factors such as cultural beliefs and practices, also hinder the delivery of quality postnatal care in SSA [18, 35]. Many women in the region follow traditional birthing practices, which can make it difficult for healthcare workers to provide the care that is needed [35]. Additionally, there may be cultural taboos surrounding certain aspects of postnatal care, such as institutional childbirth, which can make it difficult for women to access PNC [33].

One of the strongest predictors of postnatal care use is women's empowerment and autonomy [41]. The evidence suggests, that living in communities where the majority of women are empowered, that is, educated and financially independent, is advantageous for access and utilization of postnatal care in sub-Saharan Africa [29]. Furthermore, women who reside in places where their freedom is curtailed, due to certain cultural beliefs or social restrictions on women and/or insecure places such as conflict situations are less likely to seek postnatal care after childbirth. Relational factors have also been shown to be significant contextual determinants of postnatal care use. These elements mostly stem from regular contacts or relationships that women have with males. These relationships may have an impact on whether or not women choose to receive maternity care. Furthermore, household size, the number of children per household, and small family norms also influence the decision to access postnatal care [41].

8. Conclusions and recommendations

Postnatal care is beneficial and essential for maternal and newborn survival, yet access and utilization of these services are still low in SSA and vary among nations. This chapter demonstrates how individual, health system and contextual factors influence postnatal care access and utilization in sub-Saharan Africa.

In summary, postnatal care in SSA is confronted with significant challenges, including a lack of access to basic healthcare services, poor infrastructure, inadequate staffing and training, and limited resources. Cultural beliefs and practices as well as socio-economic factors that hinder women's autonomy and ability to make decisions regarding their health also play a role in hindering access to quality postnatal care. These challenges, coupled with high rates of maternal and infant mortality, underscore the need for targeted interventions and resources to improve postnatal care in the region. Efforts such as empowering women socially and economically, providing education, training healthcare professionals, and building or upgrading healthcare infrastructure can help to address these challenges and improve access, quality and utilization of postnatal care for mothers and babies in sub-Saharan Africa.

The fact that a high proportion of childbirths occur outside of healthcare institutions is one of the biggest obstacles to providing postnatal care in sub-Saharan Africa [37]. To address this challenge, postnatal care services must be made available in a vicinity near the home or at home, especially for women who give birth outside of medical facilities [14]. This is particularly important in communities where access to early postnatal care is restricted by cultural, socioeconomic, and geographic constraints. Currently, WHO and UNICEF, through the "Every Woman and Newborn" Initiative [5] are supporting countries to strengthen their routine health information systems to capture information on "early routine postnatal care utilization" (within 2 days of birth), to facilitate the achievement of the global target of 80% coverage of "early postnatal care" and national target of 90% of countries with >60% coverage [42]. Increasing coverage of skilled birth attendance is also likely to impact uptake of PNC significantly within the SSA region.

To accelerate progress in reaching the SDG global targets, it is essential to promote the completion of the maternal and newborn continuum of care, which includes care during the postnatal period, especially within 2 days after birth, due to the vital role of care during this period in improving the survival of mothers and their babies [5]. It is also essential to attain high-quality postnatal care with equity in all countries. Such efforts are likely to improve health outcomes for women and children and contribute to achieving sustainable development goals (2030).

Acknowledgements

We acknowledge the support of the WHO HRP Alliance (UNDP-UNFPA-WHO-World Bank) Special Programme for Research and Training in Human Reproduction (HRP), a co-sponsored programme executed through the University of Ghana School of Public Health, in the preparation and dissemination of this review.

Conflict of interest

The authors declare no conflict of interest.

Author details

Juliana Yartey Enos[1*], Richard Dickson Amoako[2], Samuel Kweku Enos[3], Beatrice Hayford[1] and Edem Magdalene Tette[4]

1 Department of Epidemiology, Noguchi Memorial Institute for Medical Research, College of Health Sciences, University of Ghana, Accra, Ghana

2 Department of Educational Leadership and Policy Studies, College of Education, Health and Human Development, University of Tennessee, Knoxville, Tennessee, United States of America

3 Department of Community Health, Accra College of Medicine, Accra, Ghana

4 Department of Community Health, College of Health Sciences, University of Ghana Medical School, Accra, Ghana

*Address all correspondence to: jenos@ug.edu.gh

IntechOpen

© 2023 The Author(s). Licensee IntechOpen. This chapter is distributed under the terms of the Creative Commons Attribution License (http://creativecommons.org/licenses/by/3.0), which permits unrestricted use, distribution, and reproduction in any medium, provided the original work is properly cited.

References

[1] World Health Organization (WHO). Recommendations on Maternal and Newborn Care for a Positive Postnatal Experience. Geneva: World Health Organization; 2022. ISBN: 978 92 4 004598 9

[2] Lawn JE, Cousens S, Zupan J. 4 million neonatal deaths: When? Where? Why? The Lancet. 2005;**365**(9462):891-900. DOI: 10.1016/s0140-6736(05)71048-5

[3] Symonds NE, Vidler M, Wiens MO, et al. Risk factors for postpartum maternal mortality and hospital re-admission in low- and middle-income countries: A systematic review. BMC Pregnancy and Childbirth. 2023;**23**(1):303

[4] WHO. Strategies toward Ending Preventable Maternal Mortality (EPMM). Geneva, Switzerland: World Health Organization; 2015. ISBN: 978 92 4 150848 3

[5] UNICEF & WHO. Ending Preventable Newborn Deaths and Stillbirths by 2030: Moving faster towards High-Quality Universal Health Coverage in 2020-2025. New York: UNICEF; 2020

[6] United Nations Department of Economic and Social Affairs. Sustainable Development: The 17 Goals. New York, United Nations; 2015. Available from: https://sdgs.un.org/goals

[7] Menendez C, Nhampossa T, Gbeasor-Komlanvi DF, de Lauwerier VB, Gupta G, Bustreo F. Stalled global progress on preventable maternal deaths needs renewed focus and action. BMJ. 2023;**381**:1473. DOI: 10.1136/bmj.p1473

[8] United Nations Inter-Agency Group for Child Mortality Estimation (UN IGME). Levels and Trends in Child Mortality: Report 2020. Estimates Developed by the United Nations Inter-Agency Group for Child Mortality Estimation. New York: United Nations Children's Fund; 2020 ISBN: 978-92-806-5147-8

[9] Wehrmeister FC, Faye CB, da Silva ICM, et al. Wealth- related inequalities in reproductive, maternal, newborn and child health interventions coverage among sub-Saharan African countries. Bulletin of the World Health Organization. 2020;**98**(6):394-405

[10] WHO, UNICEF, UNFPA, The World Bank Group and the United Nations Population Division. Trends in Maternal Mortality: 2000 to 2020. Geneva: WHO; 2023 Available from: https://www.who.int/publications/i/item/9789240068759

[11] World Health Organization. Maternal Mortality. Geneva: WHO; 2023 Available from: https://www.who.int/news-room/fact-sheets/detail/maternal-mortality

[12] Hug L, Alexander M, You D, et al. National, regional, and global levels and trends in neonatal mortality between 1990 and 2017, with scenario-based projections to 2030: A systematic analysis. The Lancet Global Health. 2019;7(6):e710-e720

[13] Countdown to 2030 collaboration. Countdown to 2030: Tracking progress towards universal coverage for reproductive, maternal, newborn, and child health. Lancet. 2018;**391**:1538-1548

[14] World Health Organization. Home Visits for the Newborn Child: A Strategy to Improve Survival. WHO/UNICEF Joint Statement. Geneva: WHO; 2009

Available from: https://apps.who.int/iris/handle/10665/70002

[15] Darmstadt GL, Bhutta ZA, Cousens S, Adam T, Walker N, de Bernis L. Evidence-based, cost-effective interventions: How many newborn babies can we save? Lancet. 2005;**365**(9463):977-988. DOI: 10.1016/s0 140-6736(05)71088-6

[16] Darmstadt GL, Hassan M, Balsara ZP, Winch PJ, Gipson R, Santosham M. Impact of clean delivery-kit use on newborn umbilical cord and maternal puerperal infections in Egypt. Journal of Health, Population, and Nutrition. 2009;**27**(6):746-754

[17] Wigley AS, Tejedor-Garavito N, Alegana V, Carioli A, Ruktanonchai CW, Pezzulo C, et al. Measuring the availability and geographical accessibility of maternal health services across sub-Saharan Africa. BMC Medicine. 2020;**18**:237. DOI: 10.1186/s12916-020-01707-6

[18] Kyei-Nimakoh M, Carolan-Olah M, McCann TV. Access barriers to obstetric care at health facilities in sub-Saharan Africa: A systematic review. Systematic Reviews. 2017;**6**:110. DOI: 10.1186/s13643-017-0503-x

[19] Amouzou A, Ziqi M, Carvajal-Aguirre L, et al. Skilled attendant at birth and newborn survival in sub-Saharan Africa. Journal of Global Health. 2017;**7**(2):020504-020604

[20] Sidze EM, Wekesah FM, Kisia L, Abajobir A. Inequalities in access and utilization of maternal, Newborn and child health services in sub-Saharan Africa: A special focus on urban settings. Maternal and Child Health Journal. 2022;**26**(2):250-279

[21] Faye CM, Wehrmeister FC, Melesse DY, et al. Large and persistent subnational inequalities in reproductive, maternal, newborn and child health intervention coverage in sub-Saharan Africa. BMJ Global Health. 2020;**5**(1):e002232

[22] Barros AJD, Ronsmans C, Axelson H, et al. Equity in maternal, newborn, and child health interventions in countdown to 2015: A retrospective review of survey data from 54 countries. The Lancet. 2012;**379**(9822):1225-1233

[23] Tessema ZT, Yazachew L, Tesema GA, Teshale AB. Determinants of postnatal care utilization in sub-Saharan Africa: A meta and multilevel analysis of data from 36 sub-Saharan African countries. Italian Journal of Pediatrics. 2020;**46**(1):175. DOI: 10.1186/s13052-020-00944-y

[24] Birmeta K, Dibaba Y, Woldeyohannes D. Determinants of maternal health care utilization in Holeta town, Central Ethiopia. BMC Health Services Research. 2013;**13**:256. DOI: 10.1186/1472-6963-13-256

[25] Yebyo H, Alemayehu M, Kahsay A. Why do women deliver at home? Multilevel modelling of Ethiopian National Demographic and health survey data. PLoS One. 2015;**10**(4):e0124718

[26] Galaa SZ, Daare K. Understanding barriers to maternal child health services utilization in northern Ghana. Journal of Social Development in Africa. 2008;**23**(2):127-155

[27] Gabrysch S, Cousens S, Cox J, Campbell OM. The influence of distance and level of care on delivery place in rural Zambia: A study of linked national data in a geographic information system. PLOS Medicine. 2011;**8**(1):e1000394

[28] Kruk ME, Hermosilla S, Larson E, Vail D, Chen Q, Mazuguni F, et al. Who is left behind on the road to universal facility delivery? A cross-sectional multilevel analysis in rural Tanzania.

Tropical Medicine & International Health. 2015;**20**(8):1057-1066

[29] Simona S, Lumamba C, Moyo F, Ng'andu E. The influence of contextual factors on maternal healthcare utilization in sub-Saharan Africa: A scoping review of multilevel models. Preprint medRxiv. 2022;**10**(3):2-31. DOI: 10.1101/2022.03.15.22272437

[30] Kruk ME, Rockers PC, Mbaruku G, Paczkowskie MM, Galea S. Community and health system factors associated with facility delivery in rural Tanzania: A multilevel analysis. Health Policy. 2010;**97**(2-3):209-216

[31] Say L, Raine R. A systematic review of inequalities in the use of maternal health care in developing countries: Examining the scale of the problem and the importance of context. Bulletin World Health Organisation. 2007;**85**(10):812-819

[32] Lang-Balde R, Amerson R. Culture and birth outcomes in sub-Saharan Africa: A review of literature. Journal of Transcultural Nursing. 2018;**29**(5):465-472

[33] Moyer CA, Adongo PB, Aborigo RA, Hodgson A, Engmann C, DeVries R. "It's up to the Woman's people": How social factors influence facility-based delivery in rural northern Ghana. Maternal and Child Health. 2014;**18**(1):109-119

[34] Kohi TW, Mselle LT, Dol J, Aston M. When, where and who? Accessing health facility delivery care from the perspective of women and men in Tanzania: A qualitative study. BMC Health Services Research. 2018;**18**:564

[35] Dahab R, Sakellariou D. Barriers to accessing maternal care in low-income countries in Africa: A systematic review. International Journal of Environmental Research and Public Health. 2020;**17**(12):4292

[36] Stephenson R, Baschieri A, Clements S, Hennink M, Madise N. Contextual influences on the use of health facilities for childbirth in Africa. American Journal of Public Health. 2006;**96**(1):84-93

[37] Warren C. "Postnatal care," in opportunities for Africa's Newborns: Practical data, policy and programmatic support for newborn care in Africa. In: Lawn J, Kerber K, editors. WHO on Behalf of the Partnership for Maternal, Newborn, and Child Health. Geneva: WHO; 2006

[38] Oduse S, Temesgen Z, North D. Decomposing the urban–rural inequalities in the utilisation of maternal health care services: Evidence from 27 selected countries in sub-Saharan Africa. Reproductive Health. 2021;**18**(1):1-216

[39] WHO\UNFPA\UNICEF. Reduction of Maternal Mortality: A Joint WHO/UNFPA/ UNICEF/World Bank Statement. Geneva: WHO; 2019

[40] Girum T, Wasie A. Correlates of maternal mortality in developing countries: An ecological study in 82 countries. Maternal Health, Neonatology and Perinatology. 2017;**3**:19. DOI: 10.1186/s40748-017-0059-8

[41] Mohan D, Gupta S, LeFevre A, Bazant E, Killewo J, Baqui AH. Determinants of postnatal care use at health facilities in rural Tanzania: Multilevel analysis of a household survey. BMC Pregnancy and Childbirth. 2015;**15**:282

[42] Chou AL, Hogan D, Zhang S, Moller AB, Gemmill A, et al. Global, regional, and national levels and trends in maternal mortality between 1990 and 2015, with scenario-based projections to 2030: A systematic analysis by the UN maternal mortality estimation inter-agency group. Lancet. 2016;**387**(10017):462-474